STUDENT WORKBOOK TO ACC

NURSING ASSISTANT

A Nursing Process Approach

8th Edition

Barbara R. Hegner, MSN, RN

Professor Emerita
Nursing and Life Science
Long Beach City College (CA)

Delmar Publishers

an International Thomson Publishing company I**T**P®

Albany • Bonn • Boston • Cincinnati • Detroit • London • Madrid
Melbourne • Mexico City • New York • Pacific Grove • Paris • San Francisco
Singapore • Tokyo • Toronto • Washington

NOTICE TO THE READER

COPYRIGHT © 1999
By Delmar Publishers

an International Thomson Publishing company I(T)P®

The ITP logo is a trademark under license
Printed in the United States of America

For more information contact:

Delmar Publishers
3 Columbia Circle, Box 15015
Albany, New York 12212-5015

International Thomson Publishing Europe
Berkshire House
168-173 High Holborn
London, WC1V7AA
United Kingdom

Nelson ITP, Australia
102 Dodds Street
South Melbourne,
Victoria, 3205 Australia

Nelson Canada
1120 Birchmont Road
Scarborough, Ontario
M1K 5G4, Canada

International Thomson Publishing France
Tour Maine-Montparnasse
33 Avenue du Maine
75755 Paris Cedex 15, France

International Thomson Editores
Seneca 53
Colonia Polanco
11560 Mexico D. F. Mexico

International Thomson Publishing GmbH
Königswinterer Strasße 418
53227 Bonn
Germany

International Thomson Publishing Asia
60 Albert Street
#15-01 Albert Complex
Singapore 189969

International Thomson Publishing Japan
Hirakawa-cho Kyowa Building, 3F
2-2-1 Hirakawa-cho, Chiyoda-ku,
Tokyo 102, Japan

ITE Spain/ Paraninfo
Calle Magallanes, 25
28015-Madrid, Espana

Printed in the United States of America

2 3 4 5 6 7 8 9 10 XXX   03   02   01   00   99   98

ISBN: 0-8273 9062-9

Library of Congress Card Number: 98-9510

Contents

To The Learner

The content of this workbook follows a basic organizational plan. Each lesson in the workbook includes:

■ behavioral objectives

■ a summary of the related unit in the *Nursing Assistant* text

■ exercises to help you review, recall, and reinforce concepts that have been taught

■ Nursing Assistant Alerts, which are key points to remember about each unit. The Alerts are reminders of the important concepts of the unit and the benefits to be obtained from them.

■ opportunities to apply nursing assistant care to the nursing process and expand your horizons

It has been shown that students who complete a special guide as they learn new materials perform better, have greater confidence, and are more secure in the basic concepts than those who do not.

You may wish to complete the workbook activities in preparation for your class, or after, while the information is fresh in your mind. In either case, the workbook and class work will reinforce each other.

You can make the best use of the workbook if you:

■ Read and study the related chapter in the text.

■ Observe and listen carefully to your instructor's explanations and demonstrations.

■ Read over the behavioral objectives before you start the workbook and then check to be sure you have met them after completion of the lesson exercises.

■ Use the summary to review the chapter content.

■ Complete the activities in the workbook. Circle any questions you are unable to finish to discuss with your instructor at the next class meeting.

It is the author's sincere desire that the workbook will offer you support as you learn to become the best nursing assistant.

You have chosen a special goal for yourself. You have decided to become a knowledgeable, skilled nursing assistant. Keep this goal in mind, but realize that to reach it, you need to take many small steps. Each step you master takes you closer to your ultimate goal.

Barbara R. Hegner

Tips on Studying Effectively

THE LEARNING PROCESS

Students may feel anxious about the learning process. However, learning really can be pleasurable and rewarding if you have an open mind, a desire to succeed, and a willingness to follow some simple steps.

You already have won half the battle because you have entered a training program. This shows your desire to accomplish a real life goal: to become a nursing assistant.

Steps to Learning

There are three basic steps to learning:
- Active listening
- Effective studying
- Careful practicing

Active Listening

Listening actively is not easy, natural or passive. It is, however, a skill that can be learned. Good listeners are not born, they are made. Studies show the average listening efficiency in this culture is only about 25 percent. That means that although you may hear (a passive action) all that is being said, you actually listen to and process only about one-quarter of the material. Effective listening requires a conscious effort by listeners. The most neglected communication skill is listening.

An important part of your work as a nursing assistant involves active listening to patients and coworkers. To learn this skill properly, you must begin to listen actively to your instructor or supervisor. Hearing but not processing information puts you and your patient in jeopardy.

Active listening is listening with personal involvement. There are three actions in active listening:
- Hearing what is said (passive action)
- Processing the information (active action)
- Using the information (active action)

Hearing what is said. People speak at an average rate of 125 words per minute. You must pay close attention to the speaker to hear what is said. This is not a difficult task if you do not let other thoughts and sounds interfere with your thinking. If you sit up straight and lean forward in the classroom or stand erect in the clinical area, your whole body is more receptive. Position yourself where you can adequately see or hear and keep your attention focused on the speaker. Make eye contact if possible and remain alert.

Many distractions can break your concentration unless you take action to prevent them from doing so. For example, distractions may be:
- Interruptions such as other activities in the classroom or in the patient's unit that catch your attention or create noise.
- Daydreaming and thinking about personal activities or problems.

■ Physical fatigue; sleep and rest are powerful influences on the ability to concentrate.

■ Lack of interest because you cannot immediately see the importance of the information.

To be an effective listener, you must actively work at eliminating these distractions. You must put energy into staying focused.

Processing the information. Remember that hearing the words is not enough. You must actively process (make sense of) the words in your brain. You must put meaning to them, and that takes effort. There are things you can do to help the process. These include:

■ Interact with the speaker with eye contact, smiles, and nods.

■ Ask meaningful questions. Contribute your own comments if it is a discussion.

■ Take notes.

These actions allow your memory to establish relationships to previously learned knowledge and to make new connections.

Taking notes gives you another way to imprint what you are processing. You are not only hearing the sounds of the words but can see the important ones on paper. Notetaking helps you recall points that you may have forgotten.

Notetaking is a skill that can be learned and, if used, will improve the learning process. You may need to take notes in class, during demonstrations, and when your supervisor or instructor gives you a clinical assignment. Here are some hints to make developing this skill easier.

■ Come prepared with a pencil and paper.

■ Don't try to write down every word.

■ Write down only the important points or key words.

■ Learn to take notes in an outline form.

■ Listen with particular care to the beginning sentence. It usually reveals the primary purpose.

■ Pay special attention to the final statement. It is often a summary.

Outlines include the important points summarized in a meaningful way. Be sure to leave room so that you can add material.

There are different ways of outlining. One way is to use letters and numbers to designate important points. Another is to draw a pattern of lines to show relationships. Use either way or one of your own design, but be consistent. Practice helps you master the skill of outlining.

As you make notes of material that is not clear, add a star or some other mark next to the material. When the speaker asks for questions, you can quickly find yours.

If the speaker stresses a point, be sure to mark your outline by underlining the information. This will call special attention to the points when you use the outline for study.

After class you can reorganize your notes and compare them to your text readings.

General tips

Here are some general tips to help you study better.

■ Feel certain that each lesson you master is important to prepare your knowledge and skills. The workbook, text, and instructor materials have been carefully coordinated to meet the objectives. Review the objectives before you begin to study. They are like a road map that will take you to your goal.

■ Remember that you are the learner, so you can take credit for your success. The instructor is an important guide and the workbook, text, and clinical experiences are tools, but you are the learner and whether you use the tools wisely is finally up to you.

■ Take an honest look at yourself and your study habits. Take positive steps to avoid habits that could limit your success. For example, do you let family responsibilities or social opportunities interfere with study times? If so, sit down with your family and plan a schedule for study that they will support and to which you ill adhere. Find a special place to study that is free from distraction. If the telephone interferes, take it off the hook or let everyone know that this is your study time.

The study plan

Plan a schedule for study. Actually sit down and write out a weekly schedule hour by hour so that you know exactly how your time is being spent. Then plan specific study time, but be realistic. Study has to be balanced with the other activities of your life. Learn to budget your time so that you have time to prepare and study on a regular basis and block in extra time when tests are scheduled. Don't forget to block in time for fun as well. Look back over the week to see how well you have kept to your schedule. If you have had difficulty, try to adjust the schedule to better meet your needs. If you have been successful, pat yourself on your back. You have done very well.

Make your study area special. It need not be elaborate, but make sure there is ample light. You should have a desk to work on and a supply of paper and pencils. Sharpen your pencils at the end of each study period and leave papers readily at hand. You may think this sounds strange, but often time is wasted at the beginning of a study session finding paper and sharpening pencils. If these things are ready when you first sit down, you can get started without distractions. Keep your medical dictionary in your work area. When you arrive at home, put your text and workbook there also. In other words, your work area should be designed for study. When you treat it this way, you will find that as soon as you sit down there, you will be psychologically prepared to study.

Class study

Now that you have your study area and work schedule organized, you need to think about how you can get the most out of your class experience.

- First, come prepared. Read the behavioral objectives and the lesson before class. This prepares you by acquainting you with the focus of the lesson and the vocabulary.

- Listen actively as the instructor explains the lesson. Keep your mind on what the instructor is saying. If your thoughts start to wander, refocus immediately.

- Take notes on the special points that are stressed. Use these as you study at home.

- Participate in class discussions. Remember that discussion subjects are chosen because they relate to the lesson. You can learn much from hearing the comments of others and by contributing your own. Pay attention to slides/films and overhead transparencies, because these offer a visual approach to the subject matter. You might even take notes on important points during a film or jot down questions you would like the instructor to answer.

- Ask intelligence and pertinent questions. Make sure your questions are simple and centered on the topic. Focus on one point at a time and jot down the answers for later review.

- Use models and charts that are available. Study them and see how they apply to the lesson.

- Carefully observe the demonstrations your instructor gives. Note in your book any change that may have been made in the procedure steps in order to conform with the policy of your facility.

- Perform return demonstrations carefully in the classroom. Remember, you are learning skills that will be used with real patients in the clinical situation.

After class

When class is over and you have had a break, you are ready to settle down and study. You can gain the most from the experience by:

- Studying in your prepared study area. Everything is ready and waiting for you if you followed the first part of this plan.

- Read over the lesson beginning with the behavioral objectives.

- Read with a highlighter or pencil in hand so you can underline or highlight important material.

- Answer the questions at the unit end. Check any you found difficult by reviewing that section of the text.

- Complete the related workbook unit.

- Review the behavioral objectives at the beginning of the unit. Ask yourself if you have met them. If not, go back and review. Prepare the next day's lesson by reading over the next day's unit.

- Use the medical dictionary for words you may learn that are not in the text glossary. The dictionary provides pronunciations.

Study groups

Studying with someone else who is trying to learn the same material can be very helpful and supportive, but there are some pitfalls you must be careful to avoid. If studying with someone else is to be effective and productive:

- Limit the number of people studying to a maximum of three; one other person is best.

- Keep focused on the subject. Don't begin to talk about classmates or the day's social events.

- Come prepared for the study session. Have your work completed. Use the study session to reinforce your learnings and explore deeper understanding of the material.

- Ask each other questions about the materials.

- Make a list of ideas to ask your instructor.

- Limit the study session to a specific length. Follow the plan and success is yours.

Study Skills

OBJECTIVES

As a result of this unit, you will be able to:

- Spell and define terms.
- Describe the effect of study skills on successful learning.
- Write the steps involved in active listening.
- List interferences to effective listening.
- Use two techniques of notetaking.
- Name ways to improve study habits.
- Effectively use the text book.

UNIT SUMMARY

Developing effective study habits can be important to a lifetime of learning. A few simple steps can make the process easier.

- Be familiar with your text. It will save time in locating information.
- Practice the steps to learning by being an active listener.
- Take notes for reference and study.
- Plan study times and practice in ways that promote learning.

ACTIVITIES

Vocabulary Exercise. Define the words in the spaces provided.

1. active listening _____
2. end unit materials_____
3. processing_____
4. behavioral objectives_____
5. glossary_____

Completion. Complete the statements in the spaces provided.

6. Behavioral objectives help to direct your _____ .
7. There are three basic steps to learning: _____ , _____ , _____ .
8. Daydreaming can _____ with your ability to listen actively.
9. Planning a schedule of classes and other responsibilities will help you use study time more _____ .
10. Use the _____ to learn the meaning of new terms and words.

11. Follow the maze. Which path will you travel?

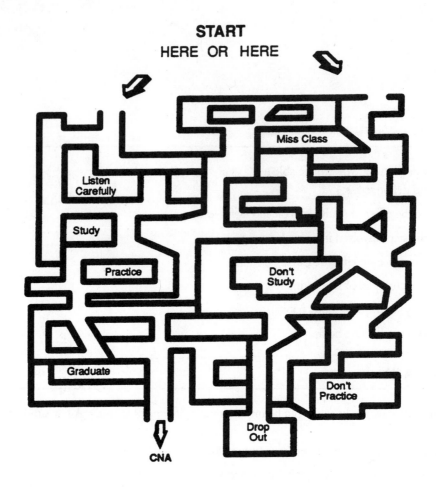

12. Name techniques of notetaking.

    a. _____

    b. _____

13. Read the case history below. Then use one or the other of the two notetaking techniques to outline the material.

Victoria Bohn was 8-1/2 months pregnant when she first appeared at our family planning clinic. The mother of three lively little girls, ages 13 months, 2 years, and 3 years, she looked tired as her children pulled at her skirts and fussed.

When her turn came to be examined, the nursing assistant found her blood pressure was 148/100, pulse 92, resp 24, temp 103°F. Her hands and fingers were swollen, and she complained of pain in her abdomen high on the right side. She had gained thirty-eight pounds since becoming pregnant. Concerned, the nursing assistant called her to the registered nurse's attention.

After examining her and listening to her baby's heartbeat, Mrs. Edelson, the registered nurse supervising the clinic, told Ms. Bohn that she wanted her to be seen by the physician.

When the physician made his examination, he immediately recommended that Ms. Bohn be admitted to the acute care facility.

During her hospitalization it was found that the patient had a severe infection in her abdomen, which was successfully treated with antibiotics. While in the hospital her blood pressure and fluid levels were brought within normal limits.

Ms. Bohn remained in the hospital until delivery of a beautiful 8-pound girl. A grandmother, who had been helping take care of the family, agreed to remain in the home for a period of time until Ms.. Bohn was once again able to manage her family herself.

Health care facilities provide health care to members of the community.

■ Specific care is provided in different types of facilities.

■ Nursing assistants play an important role in this caregiving.

■ Many changes have occurred within the last few years, brought about by increasing aging, new technologies, and the need to contain costs.

■ Different workers work as a team in departments to meet the community's health needs.

PART 1

Student Activities

SECTION 1   INTRODUCTION TO NURSING ASSISTING

UNIT 1   Community Health Care

OBJECTIVES

As a result of this unit, you will be able to:

- Spell and define terms.
- List the five basic functions of health care facilities.
- Describe four changes that have taken place in health care in the last few years.
- Describe the differences between short-term care and long-term care.
- Name the departments within a hospital.
- Describe the functions of the departments within a hospital.
- Explain three ways by which health care costs are paid.

UNIT SUMMARY

Health Care facilities provide health care to members of the community.

- Specific care is provided in different types of facilities.
- Nursing assistants play an important role in this care giving.
- Many changes have occurred within the last few years brought about by increasing aging, new technologies and the need to contain costs.
- Different workers work as a team in departments to meet the communities health needs.

ACTIVITIES

Vocabulary Exercise. Define the words in the spaces provided.

1. facility_____

2. hospice _____

3. patient _____

4. pediatric _____

5. community_____

Completion. Complete the statements in the spaces provided.

6. List five basic functions of all health care facilities.

a. _____

b. _____

c. _____

d. _____

e. _____

7. Patient focused care means _____

8. The cost of health care has increased because of demand for services as a result of _____

9. The person receiving care in an acute hospital is called a _____

10. List three examples of health care facilities.

    a. _____

    b. _____

    c. _____

11. Three names applied to the person receiving care are

    a. _____

    b. _____

    c. _____

12. Explain what activities take place in each of the following departments.

    a. Pharmacy_____

    b. Medical _____

    c. Radiology_____

    d. Pediatric_____

    e. Physical therapy _____

13. Explain the activities in each of the following departments.

    a. Dietary_____

    b. Housekeeping _____

    c. Maintenance _____

    d. Business_____

14. List four ways volunteers help patients.

    a. _____

    b. _____

    c. _____

    d. _____

15. The majority of health care is paid for with _____

Word Search.

16. Find the following words in the puzzle. Put a circle around each word and define each in the spaces provided.

    a. hospice_____

    b. postpartum _____

    c. prenatal _____

    d. pathology_____

    e. facility _____

```
Q W N B V T C R H T G N D P T N V P O L D O X C M I V M P
N J P R H Z U P W I Y L Y W L G Y A Q Y H X I X P K E X A
O W D S E X J O X A N U B Q C W O T I E X A V N D X O I L
H N A T U O P S U O S Y D J E T K H T M X L F R V G S D F
D S O V J B L T I E Q P Z R K Z B O T F C W A X M P C O M
R I S C N P N P S K F R N K D T M L P V O G C L S G L I Z
H E A L T H M A I N T E N A N C E O R G A N I Z A T I O N
O V P Q U J U R C W S N L E V R N G T I Q S L P K H E W O
S H I N E V J T Q H W A R H P O Y Y C X A L I V C U N Q P
P H O R A Q I U T C U T N X A J C O N K S I T E I K T S B
I G D S E N Q M R G E A L N X Q B H Q D G Z Y T A P U H U
C I B S K V L I J D P L H K D U N S F P L T I U K S B I E
E B L N L Z G T M U K O X D X M L S G T N P P H O I P U D
```

DEVELOPING GREATER INSIGHT

17. Visit a local community health agency such as the Health Department and learn about its services. Report back to the class.

18. Accompany a volunteer in a hospital. Learn about the volunteer's work and see how many departments you can identify.

19. Make a list of the health care facilities within your immediate vicinity and identify the type of care provided in each.

20. Invite a nursing assistant employed by a health care facility to visit the class and discuss the care provided by nursing assistants.

UNIT 2   Role of the Nursing Assistant

OBJECTIVES

As a result of this unit, you will be able to:
- Spell and define terms.
- Identify the members of the interdisciplinary health care team.
- Identify the members of the nursing team.
- List the job responsibilities of the nursing assistant.
- Make a chart showing the lines of authority an assistant follows.
- List the rules of personal hygiene and explain the importance of a healthy mental attitude.
- Describe the appropriate dress for the job.
- Describe the importance of good human relationships.
- List the ways to build productive working relationships with staff members.

UNIT SUMMARY

The nursing assistant:
- Has specific responsibilities that vary within different agencies, but must always function within the scope of nursing assistant practice.
- Must follow established procedures and policies.
- Represents herself or himself and the agency. Good grooming is essential.
- Is ultimately responsible for his or her own actions.
- Must develop good interpersonal relationships with patients, visitors, and coworkers. This will help the nursing assistant to be more effective.
- Will find that personal adjustment is made easier by understanding and obeying hospital policies and procedures. Also, that patients, coworkers, and visitors must be treated with dignity.
- Must take a written or oral and clinical test to be certified.
- May be cross-trained to increase his or her skills.

NURSING ASSISTANT ALERT

Action	Benefit
Maintain good grooming.	Enhances appearance and health. Inspires patient confidence.
Make sure uniform is complete.	Identifies your role and responsibilities.
Practice stress reduction.	Keeps you mentally and emotionally stable.

ACTIVITIES

Vocabulary Exercise. Define the words in the spaces provided.

1. attitude _____

2. burnout _____

3. nursing team _____

4. scope of practice _____

5. nursing assistant _____

Completion. Complete the statements in the spaces provided.

6. Write four terms used to describe the nursing assistant.

   a. _____

   b. _____

   c. _____

   d. _____

7. List three members of the nursing team.

   a. _____

   b. _____

   c. _____

8. Explain what is meant by the "line of authority."

   _____

   _____

9. What should you do if you have any doubts about your assignment?

   _____

10. State the three primary ways nursing care is organized and give a brief explanation of each.

    a. primary nursing _____

    _____

    b. functional nursing _____

    _____

    c. team nursing _____

    _____

11. List three goals of patient focused care.

    a. _____

    b. _____

    c. _____

12. Name three characteristics of a successful nursing assistant.

    a. _____

    b. _____

    c. _____

13. List three activities you could carry out to ensure good personal hygiene.

    a. _____

    b. _____

    c. _____

14. Explain why wearing jewelry is unwise when you are on duty.

    _____

    _____

15. What jewelry is part of your uniform?

    _____

16. The main concern of every nursing assistant should be the well-being and

    _____

17. List four reasons why a patient might be irritable, complaining, or uncooperative.

    a. _____

    b. _____

    c. _____

    d. _____

18. What are the three-dimensional aspects of a human being?

    a. _____

    b. _____

    c. _____

19. List five ways you can ensure good working relationships.

    a. _____

    b. _____

    c. _____

    d. _____

    e. _____

20. Check the positive and negative grooming traits of a nursing assistant.

Trait	Yes	No
a. long hair		
b. clean shoelaces		
c. cigarette odor		
d. bright nail polish		
e. unpolished shoes		
f. dangling earrings		
g. light lipstick		
h. long fingernails		
i. use of antiperspirant/deodorant		

21. Explain why stress is a factor for all nursing assistants and how you can reduce its effects.

_____

_____

_____

22. Define:

   a. Multiskilled worker _____

   b. Cross-training _____

23. Complete the chart to demonstrate the proper lines of communications.

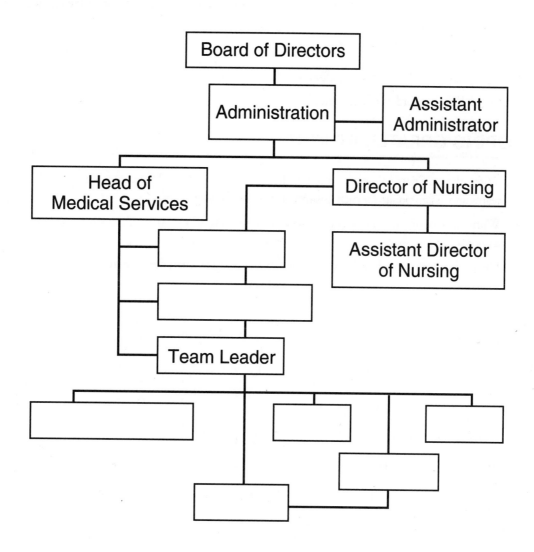

Matching. Match the specialist and the type of care provided.

Type of Care

24. _____ Care of the aging person

25. _____ Treats and diagnoses disorders of the eye.

26. _____ Treats disorders of the skin.

27. _____ Treats disorders of the digestive system.

28. _____ Treats disorders of the heart and blood vessels.

29. _____ Treats and diagnoses disorders of the nervous system.

30. _____ Treats disorders of the blood.

31. _____ Cares for women during pregnancy.

32. _____ Diagnoses and treats with x-rays.

33. _____ Treats disorders of the mind.

Specialist

a. Cardiologist

b. Gastroenterologist

c. Neurologist

d. Radiologist

e. Obstetrician

f. Hematologist

g. Psychiatrist

h. Ophthalmologist

i. Gerontologist

j. Dermatologist

DEVELOPING GREATER INSIGHT

34. With other students, role-play a properly dressed and improperly dressed nursing assistant. Divide the class into teams and assign points for each positive or negative finding.

35. With the class, discuss ways you have personally found to relieve stress. Discuss why alcohol and other drugs are a poor solution to stress.

36. Discuss burnout, what it feels like, and how people behave when they experience it. Try to learn what effect it might have on the individual, coworkers, and patients.

UNIT 3 Consumer Rights and Responsibilities in Health Care

OBJECTIVES

As a result of this unit, you will be able to:

- Spell and define terms.
- Explain the purpose of health care consumer rights.
- Describe six items that are common to Resident's Rights, the Patient's Bill of Rights, and the Client's Rights in Home Care.
- List three specific rights from each of the three documents.
- Describe eight responsibilities of health care consumers.

UNIT SUMMARY

Consumer rights are protect patients and ensure optimum care. They are spelled out in special documents such as:

- Patient's Bill of Rights.
- Client's Rights in Home Care.
- Resident's Rights.

Consumer rights are protected and optimal care is better ensured when consumers participate in the process by:

- Sharing health histories openly.
- Participating in their own care to the extent possible.
- Accepting financial responsibility.
- Being sure they understand care directions.

NURSING ASSISTANT ALERT

Action	Benefit
Understand and be guided by consumer rights	Protects patients Ensures optimal care

ACTIVITIES

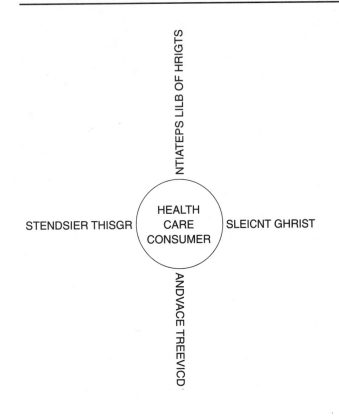

Vocabulary Exercise. Using the definitions, unscramble the words that identify documents designed to protect consumers of health care.

1. Given to patients upon admission to a hospital

2. Relates to people receiving care at home

3. Given to people before admission to long-term care

4. Gives instructions about consumers' wishes about care when they are unable to make their wishes known

Completion. Complete the following statements by using the correct term(s) from the list provided. Some may be used more than once.

accept	clarification	Client's Rights	federal
financial	honestly	medications	past
Patient's Bill of Rights	responsibility	will not	

5. The Omnibus Budget Reconciliation Act of 1987 is _____ legislation.

6. A copy of the _____ is given to people upon admission to a hospital.

7. A copy of the _____ is given to consumers during the first home visit.

8. Consumers have _____ to maintain personal health care records.

9. Consumers are responsible for communicating _____ with the physician and other caregivers.

10. It is important for consumers to provide accurate information regarding _____ hospitalizations and

_____ .

11. Consumers are responsible for informing health care providers if they _____ be able to carry out prescribed treatment.

12. Consumers must _____ responsibility for learning how to manage their health.

13. Consumers are responsible for asking for _____ if they do not fully understand instructions.

14. Consumers are responsible for assuming _____ responsibility for health care.

True/False. Mark the following true or false by circling T or F.

15. T   F   All citizens in the United States have certain rights that are guaranteed by law.

16. T   F   Consumers have no rights once they enter a health care facility.

17. T F The Omnibus Budget Reconciliation Act of 1987 was legislated by the federal government to ensure the rights of patients in acute care facilities.

18. T F Informed consent means the person gives permission for care even if he or she does not fully understand the purpose of the care.

19. T F A grievance is a situation in which the consumer feels there are grounds for a complaint.

20. T F Both caregiver and consumer have responsibilities that help ensure optimal health care.

21. T F Residents have the right to determine the cost of care.

22. T F All personal and clinical records pertaining to a patient must be kept confidential.

23. T F Unless a consumer gives consent, an experimental procedure may not be performed.

24. T F In long-term care, visitors may be restricted against the resident's wishes.

25. T F Patients have a role in decision making for treatment choices and planning of care.

26. T F Patients have the right to open and honest communication with caregivers.

27. T F A patient who feels that he has been injured must keep this information to himself.

28. T F A resident has the right to choose an attending physician.

29. T F The resident has the right to freedom from corporal punishment.

30. T F Patients must accept the treatment prescribed by their physicians.

31. T F Patients do not have the right to examine their medical bills as long as the insurance company is paying those bills.

32. T F Patients have the right to know if the physician and other health workers are in business together.

Identification. Determine the appropriateness of a nursing assistant's behavior by indicating C for correct or I for incorrect.

33. _____ Listening to visitors' conversations.

34. _____ Discussing a resident's physical status with a relative.

35. _____ Making shift reports so that patients cannot hear.

36. _____ Reading a patient's record to satisfy your curiosity.

37. _____ Sharing the medical records with the resident's minister.

38. _____ Telling a patient that his or her roommate has a terminal condition.

39. _____ Telling another nursing assistant that a resident eats best when fed from the right side.

40. _____ Sharing information with another staff member that the resident is incontinent.

41. _____ Telling another resident that a roommate has dirty toenails.

42. _____ Mentioning that a patient has beautiful white hair to his or her roommate.

43. _____ Treating patients with dignity and respect.

44. _____ Handling a patient's personal items carefully.

45. _____ Not telling the client your name before beginning care.

46. _____ Letting a patient know that someone else will be making the next visit.

47. _____ Not allowing the client to assist with a bath when he is able to do so.

48. _____ Explaining restrictions on the number of visitors each patient may have while in intensive care.

49. _____ Referring the patient's request about his blood pressure to the nurse.

50. _____ Telling the patient's daughter that her father doesn't have long to live.

UNIT 4   Ethical and Legal Issues Affecting the Nursing Assistant

OBJECTIVES

As a result of this unit, you will be able to:
- Spell and define terms.
- Discuss ethical and legal situations in health care.
- Describe the ethical responsibilities of the nursing assistant concerning patient information.
- Describe tactful ways to refuse a tip offered by a patient.
- Describe the legal responsibilities of a nursing assistant.
- Describe how to protect the patient's right to privacy.

UNIT SUMMARY

All persons giving health care voluntarily adhere to a set of ethical standards. They agree to:
- Protect life.
- Promote health.
- Keep personal information confidential.
- Respect personal death beliefs.
- Give care based on need, not gratuities (tips).
- Provide safety.

Nursing assistants have legal responsibilities. Legal situations the health care provider wants to avoid include:
- Negligence.
- Assault and battery.
- Theft.
- Invasion of privacy.
- Abuse.

NURSING ASSISTANT ALERT

Action	Benefit
Maintain ethical standards.	Protects patients' rights and privacy.
Obey laws.	Protects you against legal actions and keeps patient safe.
Carry out orders or report inability to do so to supervisor.	Ensures proper and safe nursing care
Protect patients' physical and personal privacy.	Promotes patients' sense of security. Patients feel secure and protected.

ACTIVITIES

Vocabulary Exercise. Define the words in the spaces provided.

1. confidential_____

2. assault_____

3. negligence_____

4. verbal abuse _____

5. slander _____

Completion. Complete the statements in the spaces provided.

6. Ethical standards are a _____ code rather than a legal code.

7. List four medical ethics questions under current scrutiny by the medical profession.

    a. _____

    b. _____

    c. _____

    d. _____

8. Explain how you could assure that the patient receives the proper treatment.

    _____

    _____

9. The patient offers you a tip for getting him fresh water. Describe and explain your response._____

    _____

10. You have not stolen something belonging to a patient yourself, but you observed someone else do so and failed to report the fact. Of what crime are you guilty?

    _____

11. The visitor asks you if her father really has cancer. What response should you make?

    _____

12. A physical restraint is any device that_____

_____

13. Abuse is any act that is _____ and causes harm to the patient.

14. A door that is shut against a patient's will when the patient is confined to bed is a form of_____ .

True/False. Mark the following true or false by circling T or F.

15. T   F   It is the responsibility of a nursing assistant to determine that abuse of a patient has taken place.

16. T   F   A nursing assistant who reports bruises or wounds noted on a patient is acting properly.

17. T   F   Self-abuse may occur when a disabled person is unable to adequately carry out ADLs and not accept help.

18. T   F   Signs of poor personal hygiene and a change of personality may indicate abuse.

19. T   F   Most abuse originates in feelings of frustration and fatigue.

20. T   F   For help in reducing personal stress, request counseling through an Employee Assistance Program.

21. T   F   Separation of a patient may be permitted if it is part of a therapeutic plan to reduce agitation.

22. T   F   A nursing assistant may independently decide to isolate a patient.

23. T   F   In some states a person not reporting abuse is held as guilty as the abusing person.

Complete the Chart. Place an X in the appropriate space to determine which type of abuse has taken place.

Action	Verbal Abuse	Sexual Abuse	Psychological Abuse	Physical Abuse
24. Touching a patient in a sexual way				
25. Using obscene gestures				
26. Raising your voice in anger				
27. Teasing a patient				
28. Handling a patient roughly				
29. Making threats				
30. Making fun of the patient				
31. Ridiculing patient's behavior				
32. Suggesting the patient engage in sexual acts with you				
33. Hitting a patient				

UNIT 5   Medical Terminology and Body Organization

OBJECTIVES

As a result of this unit, you will be able to:
- Spell and define terms.
- Recognize the meanings of common prefixes, suffixes, and root words.
- Build medical terms from word parts.
- Write the abbreviations commonly used in health care facilities.
- Describe the simple to complex organization of the body.
- Name four types of tissues and their characteristics.
- Name and locate major organs as parts of body systems, using proper anatomic terms.

UNIT SUMMARY

Medical terminology is developed by arranging and combining word parts. It is a language used by health personnel in health care facilities. The words are formed of:
- Word roots.
- Prefixes at the beginning of words.
- Suffixes a the end of words.
- Combining forms referring to body parts and medical actions.
- Abbreviations (usually letters).

The human body is organized into:
- Various kinds of cells.
- Four basic tissue types.
- Many organs.
- Nine systems.

Each contributes in a special way to the total structure and physiology of the body. A careful study of the healthy body and its organization provides a foundation for learning about your own body and the bodies of your patients. Learning medical terminology will improve your understanding and will help you communicate more effectively in the health care setting by more accurately reporting and documenting your observations.

NURSING ASSISTANT ALERT

Action	Benefit
Analyze medical and scientific terms	Improves comprehension. Increases vocabulary. Improves communication skills.

Action	Benefit
Practice using combining forms.	Increases verbal and written skills.
Study the anatomy and physiology of the body.	Improved understanding of normal body structure and functions.
Learn proper names for body parts.	More accurate communication of observations.

ACTIVITIES

Vocabulary Exercise. Define the words in the spaces provided.

1. prefix _____

2. suffix _____

3. abbreviation _____

4. combining forms _____

5. word root _____

Completion. Complete the statements in the spaces provided.

6. Name the book, other than your text, that would be most helpful in studying medical terms. _____

_____

7. Underline the <u>root</u> in each of the following words and give a definition of the word.

   example: <u>abdomin</u>al   pertaining to the abdomen

   a. adenoma _____

   b. colectomy _____

   c. craniotomy _____

   d. dentist _____

   e. hysterectomy _____

   f. myalgia _____

   g. nephrolithiasis _____

   h. pneumonectomy _____

   i. thoracotomy _____

   j. urinometer _____

8. Underline the <u>prefix</u> in each of the following words and give a definition of the prefix.

   example: <u>neo</u>plasm   new

   a. asepsis _____

   b. bradyeardia _____

   c. dysuria _____

   d. hypertension _____

   e. hypotension _____

f. pandemic _____

g. polyuria _____

h. gerontology _____

i. premenstrual _____

j. tachycurdia _____

9. Underline the <u>suffix</u> in each of the following words and give a definition of the suffix.

example: acro<u>megaly</u>   great

a. appendectomy _____

b. hepatitis _____

c. electrocardiogram _____

d. anemia _____

e. tracheotomy _____

f. hematology _____

g. hemiplegia _____

h. apnea _____

i. otoscope _____

j. proctoscopy _____

10. Listed below are five words not in your text. Define each and then check your accuracy with a medical dictionary.

a. adenitis _____

b. cardiopathy _____

c. leukopenia _____

d. arthroscope _____

e. cytomegaly _____

11. Substitute one word for the underlined words in each of the following statements.

example: The patient experienced <u>pus in the urine.</u>   Pyuria

a. There was <u>sugar in the urine</u>.   _____

b. The patient made an appointment with a <u>physician who specializes in female diseases</u>.   _____

c. The nurse performed a <u>puncture in</u> <u>a vein</u> and drew blood.   _____

d. The patient has an <u>incision made into the trachea</u> to ease breathing.   _____

e. The patient had a <u>tumor composed mainly of fibrous tissue</u> removed from her uterus.   _____

f. The patient was receiving chemotherapy for cancer, which caused <u>depression of all her cell levels</u>.   _____

g. The nursing assistant listened with the stethoscope to the patient's heart. She found <u>the heart rate was slow</u>.   _____

h. The medication didn't seem to help the patient's <u>high blood pressure</u>.   _____

i. The postoperative diagnosis was <u>removal of a lung</u>.   _____

j. The patient complained of pain <u>under the stomach</u>.   _____

12. Explain the following diagnoses.

a. thrombosis _____

b. pyogenic infection _____

c. pneumonitis _____

d. cystitis _____

e. mastitis _____

13. Write the name of the body part indicated by the abbreviation.

a. abd _____

b. bld _____

c. G.I. _____

d. AX _____

e. GU _____

f. vag _____

g. sh _____

Matching. Match the letters on the left with the medical diagnosis on the right.

14. _____	AIDS	a.	fracture
15. _____	CHF	b.	transient ischemic attack
16. _____	CVA	c.	infectious hepatitis
17. _____	Fx	d.	multiple sclerosis
18. _____	TIA	e.	acquired immune deficiency syndrome
19. _____	MI	f.	non-specific urethritis
20. _____	IH	g.	sexually transmitted disease
21. _____	KS	h.	cerebrovascular accident
22. _____	STD	i.	Kaposi's sarcoma
23. _____	MS	j.	myocardial infarction
		k.	congestive heart disease

Abbreviations. The following is a list of abbreviations you will find relating to orders and patient care. Write your understanding.

24. a. amb. ad lib. _____

b. urine to lab ASAP _____

c. BR only _____

d. check drg frequently _____

e. OOB daily _____

f. position HOB 45° _____

g. d/c cl liq diet _____

    h. SSE prn _____

    i. CBC in AM_____

    j. NPO preop _____

25. Write the names of the following hospital departments.

    a. CS _____

    b. EENT _____

    c. PT _____

    d. OPD _____

    e. MRD_____

    f. RR_____

    g. Peds_____

    h. DR _____

    i. OR _____

    j. Lab _____

26. Write the appropriate abbreviation for the time indicated.

    a. before meals _____

    b. twice daily _____

    c. at bedtime _____

    d. every day _____

    e. after meals _____

    f. immediately_____

    g. four times a day _____

    h. while awake _____

    i. every hour _____

    j. every other day_____

27. Write the word for each of the following measurements.

    a. $\overline{ss}$ _____

    b. mL_____

    c. lb _____

    d. kg _____

    e. > _____

Roman Numerals.

28. Write the Roman numerals for each of the following numbers.

    a. one _____

    b. twelve _____

    c. six _____

    d. nine _____

    e. four _____

29. Unscramble the medical terms and write them in the center of the star. Then define each term in the spaces provided.

a. _____

b. _____

c. _____

d. _____

e. _____

30. Complete the organizational pattern of the body.

cells → _____ → _____ → systems.

31. There are four tissue types. Write the names and give the functions.

a. _____

b. _____

c. _____

d. _____

32. Select the proper directional term from the list provided for each area indicated. Then color the organs as specified in the list.

anterior   medial

inferior   posterior

lateral   superior

Organ Colors

Appendix—brown

Liver—green

Small intestine—red

Pancreas—yellow

Stomach—orange

33. Use the correct term to identify the relationships of the body parts listed by writing the correct answer in the space provided.

			Answer
a. breasts	(anterior)	(posterior)	_____
b. heels	(anterior)	(posterior)	_____
c. toes	(anterior)	(posterior)	_____
d. buttocks	(anterior)	(posterior)	_____
e. abdomen	(anterior)	(posterior)	_____
f. breast related to legs	(superior)	(inferior)	_____
g. ankles related to legs	(superior)	(inferior)	_____
h. head related to toes	(superior)	(inferior)	_____
i. hips related to breasts	(superior)	(inferior)	_____
j. thumb related to little finger	(medial)	(lateral)	_____

34. Another term for anterior is _____.

35. Another term for posterior is _____.

36. Write the proper abbreviations for abdominal regions.

   a. Patient A is complaining of pain in the area of his appendix. You properly identify this area
   as the _____.

   b. Patient B is complaining of discomfort in the area of his stomach. You properly identify this area
   as the _____.

   c. Patient C is complaining of pain over the region of his liver. You properly identify this area
   as the _____.

   d. Patient D is complaining of pain over the region where the lower descending colon is located. You properly
   identify this area as the _____.

Matching. Place the organs in the proper systems.

Organ	System
37. _____ Spleen	a. Cardiovascular
38. _____ Brain	b. Endocrine
39. _____ Breasts	c. Digestive
40. _____ Kidneys	d. Integumentary
41. _____ Ureters	e. Skeletal
42. _____ Vagina	f. Muscular
43. _____ Bones	g. Nervous
44. _____ Heart	h. Reproductive
45. _____ Pituitary gland	i. Respiratory
46. _____ Joints	j. Urinary

Match the function and the system.

	Function		System
47. _____	Transports, absorbs food	a.	Cardiovascular
48. _____	Regulates body processes through hormones.	b.	Endocrine
49. _____	Fulfills sexual needs.	c.	Digestive
50. _____	Brings in oxygen.	d.	Integumentary
51. _____	Forms walls of some organs.	e.	Skeletal
52. _____	Eliminates liquid wastes.	f.	Muscular
53. _____	Acts as levers in movement.	g.	Nervous
54. _____	Produces hormones to regulate body functions.	h.	Reproductive
55. _____	Carries oxygen and nutrients to cells.	i.	Respiratory
56. _____	Coordinates body activities through nervous impulses.	j.	Urinary

RELATING TO THE NURSING PROCESS

Write the step of the nursing process that is related to the nursing assistant action.

Nursing Assistant Action   **Nursing Process Step**

Ex. The nursing assistant uses proper abbreviations and terms when
documenting on the patient's record.   _____Assessment_____

57. The nursing assistant reports that the patient has expressed how
fearful she is about her surgery.   _____

58. The nursing assistant accurately describes the white patches she
noted on the resident's tongue.   _____

59. The nursing assistant carries out the approaches listed on the care plan.   _____

60. The nursing assistant correctly identifies the location of the patient's pain.   _____

DEVELOPING GREATER INSIGHT

61. With a partner, find the approximate location of the following organs.

  a. brain

  b. heart

  c. lung

  d. stomach

  e. liver

  f. appendix

62. Have a partner indicate pain in some part of his or her body and then describe the area using proper anatomic terms.

63. If available, examine models such as a skeleton or torso or wall chart. Practice naming the major bones and organs.

UNIT 6   Classification of Disease

OBJECTIVES

As a result of this unit, you will be able to:
- Spell and define terms.
- Define disease and list some possible causes.
- List six major health problems.
- Identify disease-related terms.
- Distinguish between signs and symptoms.
- List ways in which a diagnosis is made.
- Describe malignant and benign tumors.

UNIT SUMMARY

Disease is any change from a healthy state. It takes many forms and has many causes. A variety of factors influences the promotion or resistance to disease. Specific terms are used when discussing disease, such as:
- Etiology.
- Signs and symptoms.
- Prognosis.
- Risk factors.
- Predisposing factors.

Major disease conditions include:
- Congenital disorders.
- Traumas.
- Chemical imbalances.
- Infections.
- Ischemias.
- Neoplasms.

Diagnosis is made using laboratory and other diagnostic tests, including:
- Ultrasound.
- Thermography.
- Magnetic resonance imaging.
- X-rays.
- Recording electrical activity of organs.
- Direct visualization procedures.

- Dye studies.
- Cardiac catheterization.

Neoplasms are common to body organs. They are:
- Benign or malignant.
- Of unknown etiology.
- Named as:
  organ plus *oma* (benign).
  sarcomas (malignant).
  carcinomas (malignant).
  special names.

Types of therapy include:
- Surgery.
- Chemotherapy.
- Radiation.
- Supportive care.

NURSING ASSISTANT ALERT

Action	Benefit
Observe signs and symptoms carefully.	Accurate information is observed.
Report observations promptly.	Prompt and proper action can be taken.

ACTIVITIES

Vocabulary Exercise. Complete the puzzle by filling in the missing letters of words found in this unit. Use the definitions to help you discover these words.

1. naming the disease process
2. protective body chemicals
3. seen by others
4. abnormalities present at birth
5. injury
6. new growths
7. treatment

1. D _ _ _ _ _ _ _ _
2. _ _ _ _ _ _ _ I _ _
3. S _ _ _ _ _
4. _ _ _ _ E _ _ _ _ _
5. _ _ A _ _ _
6. _ _ _ _ _ _ S _
7. _ _ E _ _ _ _

8. Define disease. _____

9. Define etiology. _____

Matching. Match each clinical condition with the proper pathological classification.

Condition

10. _____ fractured femur

11. _____ pneumonia

12. _____ spina bifida

13. _____ rectal abscess

14. _____ diabetes

15. _____ lupus erythematosis

16. _____ osteoma

17. _____ thrombosis

Classification

a. ischemia

b. congenital abnormalities

c. infection

d. neoplasia

e. trauma

f. inflammation

g. metabolic imbalance

h. obstruction

i. autoimmune reaction

Match the clinical condition with the common cause or predisposing factor.

Condition

18. _____ trauma

19. _____ age

20. _____ malnutrition

21. _____ tumors

22. _____ microorganisms

23. _____ radiation

24. _____ heredity

Classification

a. external

b. internal

c. predisposing

Observation

25. _____ rash

26. _____ nausea

27. _____ pain

28. _____ elevated temperature

29. _____ increased pulse rate

30. _____ vomiting

31. _____ flushed skin

32. _____ dizziness

33. _____ itching

34. _____ anxious feelings

Classification

a. sign

b. symptom

Completion. Complete the statements in the spaces provided.

35. You are assigned to the pediatric unit and have five patients in your care. Briefly explain each of their diagnoses.

    a. Jessica R has hemophilia_____

    b. Billy B has sickle cell anemia_____

    c. Jennifer F has talipes_____

    d. Casey B has cleft lip _____

    e. Leslie S has renal agenesis _____

36. Each of these cases falls into the classification of disease states known as:

    _____

37. The following week you are working in a surgical unit and find these names and diagnoses on your assignment. Define the diagnosis.

    a. Mrs. McFarland—nephroptosis_____

    b. Ms. Horton—cholelithiasis _____

    c. Mr. Hughes—renal lithiasis _____

    d. Mrs. Ramirez—cerebral thrombosis_____

38. The conditions in the previous statement involve _____ to the flow of body fluids.

39. Several of your other patients have diagnoses of metabolic imbalances. List four conditions you have learned that fall into this classification.

    a. _____

    b. _____

    c. _____

    d. _____

40. One of your patients has been admitted for surgery with a diagnosis of adenoma. You recognize this as a _____ involving a _____.

41. Mrs. Bolen is suffering from cancer of the colon. List six signs and symptoms you might note when caring for her.

    a. _____

    b. _____

    c. _____

    d. _____

    e. _____

    f. _____

42. The body has special natural defenses. List five.

    a. _____

    b. _____

    c. _____

    d. _____

    e. _____

43. List four basic forms of therapy.

a. _____

b. _____

c. _____

d. _____

Clinical Situations. Briefly describe how a nursing assistant should react to the following situation.

44. Your neighbor Elizabeth Simmons tells you she has a lump in her breast but she has told no one else.

_____

_____

_____

45. Mrs. Torres has a cerebral thrombus. Follow the maze to identify its location.

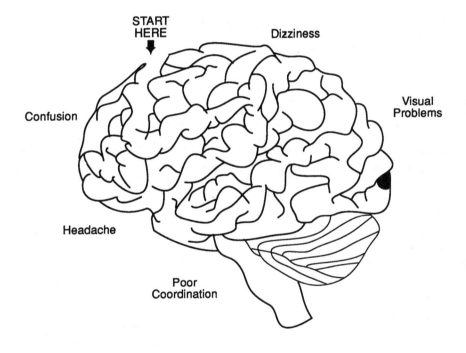

a. What part of the body is affected _____

b. Define the words:

Cerebral_____

Thrombus _____

DEVELOPING GREATER INSIGHT

46. Discuss the importance of mammograms with the class. Invite anyone who has had a mammogram to share the experience.

47. Review an unidentified case history of a person who suffered a stroke. Try to relate what you are hearing about the case to the material you have learned in this unit.

48. Discuss the use of ultrasound and MRI as diagnostic tools. Invite anyone who has experienced these tests to discuss their experience.

UNIT 7   Communication Skills

OBJECTIVES

As a result of this unit, you will be able to:

- Spell and define terms.

- Explain the types of verbal and nonverbal communication.

- Describe and demonstrate how to answer the telephone while on duty.

- Answer a patient's call signal.

- Describe four tools of communication for staff members.

- Describe the guidelines for communicating with patients with aphasia, impaired hearing, impaired vision, and disorientation.

UNIT SUMMARY

Communication is a two-way process of sharing information. Communications must be clear between yourself and patients, coworkers, and those in authority. Communications are sent through:

- Oral or verbal language.

- Body language.

- Written messages.

Special communication techniques must be used when communicating with patients with aphasia, who have impaired hearing or vision, or who are disoriented.

NURSING ASSISTANT ALERT

Action	Benefit
Communicate effectively with coworkers	Ensures that accurate information is transmitted properly. Ensures that the safest care will be given.
Communicate effectively with patients	Ensures that patients' needs will be recognized and understood. Directions will be properly understood by patients.
Communicate effectively with families and visitors	Conveys a feeling of welcome and security to family members and visitors.

ACTIVITIES

Vocabulary Exercise. Define the following by selecting the correct term from the list provided.

aphasia   body language

communication   disorientation

memo   nonverbal communication

shift report   sign language

symbols   verbal communication

1. Objects used to represent something else _____

2. A state of mental confusion _____

3. Communication with spoken words _____

4. Inability to understand spoken or written language _____

5. Report of patients and their conditions provided to the staff coming on duty by the staff of the previous shift _____

6. Communicating through body movements _____

7. Form of communication used by some hearing-impaired persons _____

8. Communicating without verbal speech _____

9. Brief communication that informs or reminds employees _____

10. Exchanging information _____

Completion. Complete the statements in the spaces provided.

11. Describe the purpose of each of the following.

   a. Employee's personnel handbook _____

   b. Disaster manual _____

   c. Procedure manual _____

   d. Nursing policy manual _____

   e. Assignment _____

12. List types of information that might be learned in a staff development class.

   a. _____

   b. _____

   c. _____

   d. _____

13. Three things are needed for successful communication. They are:

   a. _____

   b. _____

   c. _____

14. List six ways people communicate without using words.

   a. _____

   b. _____

   c. _____

   d. _____

   e. _____

   f. _____

15. State five ways you can improve communications with patients.

   a. _____

   b. _____

   c. _____

   d. _____

   e. _____

16. When you receive or give a report, what facts should be included?

   a. _____

   b. _____

   c. _____

17. List ways a message can be sent through body language.

   a. _____

   b. _____

   c. _____

   d. _____

   e. _____

   f. _____

Completion. Complete the following statements by selecting the correct term(s) from the list provided.

anger	articulate	caring	clearly	clues
cover	double	hand	happiness	hearing
identify	lengthy	lightly	loudness	objects
one	patronizing	sadness	see	slang
specific	substitutes	talking	tone	

18. When communicating verbally, remember to:

   a. Control the _____ of your voice.

   b. Control the voice _____ .

   c. Be aware of the way you _____ .

d. Avoid _____ meanings or cultural meanings.

e. Not use informal language or _____ .

19. Loudness and tone of your voice can convey a message of:

a. _____

b. _____

c. _____

d. _____

20. With a patient who is hard of hearing:

a. Make sure patient can _____ you clearly.

b. Stand on the patient's _____ side.

c. Do not _____ your mouth when speaking.

d. Speak _____ , distinctly, and naturally.

e. Use _____ gestures and body language to help express your meanings.

21. With the patient who is visually impaired:

a. Describe the environment and _____ around the patient to establish a frame of reference.

b. Touch the patient _____ on the hand to avoid startling the patient.

c. Be _____ when giving directions.

d. When entering a room, _____ yourself and your purpose.

e. Make sure patient is aware of the availability of _____ books.

22. With the disoriented patient:

a. Ask the resident to do only _____ task at a time.

b. Use word _____ if they have meaning for the patient.

c. Be specific in speech and avoid being _____ .

d. Avoid _____ explanations.

e. Use nonverbal _____ freely and respectfully.

Completion.

23. Complete the nursing organizational chart using the names presented.

rehabilitation aides   nurse manager   staff nurses

nursing assistants   unit secretaries   patient care technicians

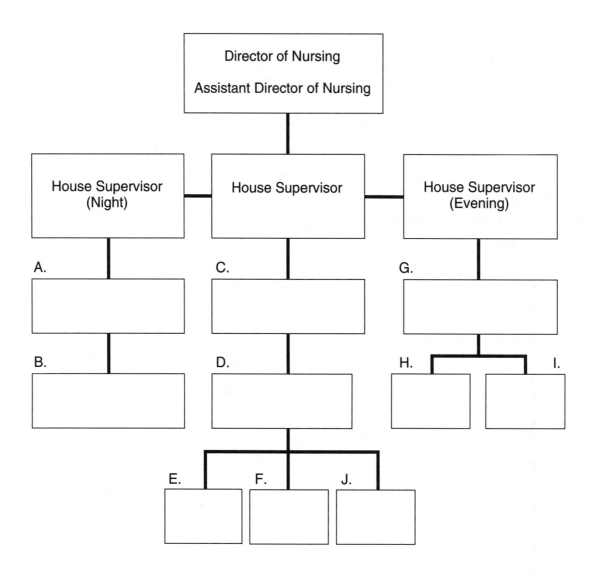

Complete the Form.

24. Father Duchene, the priest at St. Gregory's Catholic Church, called at 10:00 AM on Nov. 11th to ask how Mrs. Riley was feeling. He wanted to speak to the nurse manager, Mr. Burke, who was busy at the time and unavailable. Father Duchene asked that the nurse manager return his call. His telephone number is 683-4972. How do you communicate this information? Complete the following form to demonstrate your understanding of the proper way to do this task.

```
To                          ☐ URGENT
Date_____Time_____ A.M.
                                      P.M.
          WHILE YOU WERE OUT
From_____
Of_____
Phone_____
        Area Code        Number        Ext.
┌─────────────────┬──┬─────────────────┬──┐
│ Telephoned      │  │ Please call     │  │
├─────────────────┼──┼─────────────────┼──┤
│ Came to see you │  │ Wants to see you│  │
├─────────────────┼──┼─────────────────┼──┤
│ Returned your call│ │ Will call again │  │
└─────────────────┴──┴─────────────────┴──┘

Message _____
_____
_____
_____
_____
_____
_____
_____

Signed _____
```

Yes or No. Do the words and the body language send the same message? Indicate Yes (Y) or No (N).

25. Y   N   Wendy rubs her head with her hand and tells you she does not have a headache.

26. Y   N   Ellen sits with her arms and legs crossed, has turned her wheelchair toward the window, and tells you she is happy to meet her new daughter in law.

27. Y   N   Aimee makes a face when you feed her and says she hates chocolate pudding.

28. Y   N   Mary appears on duty with dirty shoes and untidy hair and says she is proud to be a nursing assistant.

29. Y   N   Chris keeps moving about the room and rubbing her hands together and says she feels calm about her transfer to another facility.

30. Y   N   Nichole says she is interested in her patients. She often looks out the window and seldom makes eye contact when patients speak.

31. Y   N   Carrie and Terry claim to care about patients and often talk "over" them as they work together giving care.

32. Y   N   Tim describes himself as a caring nursing assistant. He often interrupts patients when they are talking.

33. Y   N   Fernando says he is sensitive to patients' feelings and stands about two feet away when conversing with them.

34. Y   N   Grace is careful to show caring by never discussing personal activities with other staff members in the presence of patients.

Clinical Situations. Read the following situations and answer the questions.

35. Pam Bradley has been hard of hearing since she was born. A hearing aid has helped the problem, but she still occasionally uses sign language. Kate, the nursing assistant, likes to communicate with her this way.

Refer to the Figures. Interpret each picture and write the message being communicated in the space provided.

a. _____

(REPEAT MOVEMENT)

b. _____

c. _____

36. Mr. Baudine has aphasia following a stroke. You are assigned to his care. Communication with him has been particularly difficult for the staff.

   a. Describe the condition of aphasia and state a common cause.

   _____

   _____

   b. When he becomes frustrated, what action should you take?

   _____

   _____

   c. Will raising your voice help Mr. Baudine understand?

   _____

   _____

d. What are two nonverbal communication techniques that speech therapists sometimes devise to help an aphasic patient?

_____

_____

DEVELOPING GREATER INSIGHT

37. Check with your local college or deaf association and take a course in signing.

38. Practice taking messages over a telephone.

39. With your classmates, practice communicating the following messages without using words.

   a. yes, no

   b. happiness

   c. pain in the abdomen

   d. headache

   e. depression

UNIT 8   Observation, Reporting, and Documentation

OBJECTIVES

As a result of this unit, you will be able to:
- Spell and define terms.
- List the four components of the nursing process.
- Explain the responsibilities of the nursing assistant for each component of the nursing process.
- Describe two observations to make for each body system.
- Describe the purpose of the care plan.
- List three times when oral reports are given.
- Describe the information given when reporting.
- Describe the purpose of the patient's medical record.
- Explain the rules for documentation.

UNIT SUMMARY

Patient focused care is carried out most effectively when communications are accurately passed between coworkers and between caregivers and patients. This is achieved by:
- Following the nursing process.
- Developing an individual care plan for each patient.
- Proper documentation and reporting.

The nursing process has four steps and nursing assistants make a valuable contribution to each. The four steps are:
- Assessment.
- Planning.
- Implementation.
- Evaluation.

NURSING ASSISTANT ALERT

Action	Benefit
Observe carefully	Alerts nurse to changes in patient's condition so proper care can be given.
Document accurately	Keeps staff informed of patient's status.
Following nursing care plan faithfully.	Ensures proper care for the individual patient.

ACTIVITIES

Vocabulary Exercise. Each line has four different spellings of a word from this unit. Circle the correctly spelled word.

1. assesment	ascesment	accessment	assessment
2. charing	charting	sharting	chartting
3. process	procese	prosess	processe
4. graphic	grephic	grafic	graffic
5. obsavation	obserbation	observation	observachian
6. communication	comunication	cummunication	communikation
7. cardex	Kardex	cadex	kardex
8. evaleation	evaloation	evaluation	eveluation

Completion. Complete the following statements in the spaces provided.

9. The four steps of the nursing process and their definitions are:

   Step   **Definition**

   a. _____

   b. _____

   c. _____

   d. _____

10. What are three types of information you will find on the care plan?

   a. _____

   b. _____

   c. _____

11. The nursing diagnosis is a statement of _____

_____

12. The nurse coordinates assessment with _____

_____

13. The care plan is kept in the Kardex or _____

_____

14. The intervention (approach) states:

   a. _____

   b. _____

   c. _____

15. Nursing assistants are responsible for knowing when and _____ the approach is to be carried out and for implementing the approach _____ .

16. The final step in the nursing process is the _____ .

17. The nursing assistant is responsible for reporting to the nurse when _____

_____

Differentiation. Differentiate between signs and symptoms by writing each observation under the proper label in the spaces provided.

	Sign	Symptom	Observation
18.	_____	_____	nausea
19.	_____	_____	vomiting
20.	_____	_____	pain
21.	_____	_____	restlessness
22.	_____	_____	dizziness
23.	_____	_____	cold, clammy skin
24.	_____	_____	incontinence
25.	_____	_____	elevated blood pressure
26.	_____	_____	anxiety
27.	_____	_____	cough

Matching. Name the sense used to determine the following information.

28. _____ Body odor

29. _____ Radial pulse

30. _____ Wheezing when the patient breathes

31. _____ Comments from the patient

32. _____ Blood in urine

33. _____ A change in the way a patient walks

34. _____ Warmth of the patient's skin

35. _____ Bruises

36. _____ Lump under patient's skin

37. _____ The patient crying

a. eyes

b. ears

c. smell

d. touch

Matching. Match the observation on the left with the system on the right to which it best relates.

Observation

38. _____ curled up in bed

39. _____ disoriented as to time and place

40. _____ regular pulse

41. _____ elevated blood pressure

42. _____ jaundiced skin

43. _____ skin warm to touch

44. _____ difficulty breathing

45. _____ unable to respond with words

46. _____ cloudy urine

47. _____ site of injection hot and red

System

a. circulatory

b. integumentary

c. muscular

d. skeletal

e. nervous

f. respiratory

g. digestive

h. endocrine

i. reproductive

j. urinary

48. _____ difficulty passing stool

49. _____ belching frequently following meal

50. _____ vaginal discharge

51. _____ drowsy, not responding well

52. _____ nauseated, vomited small amount of clear fluid

Multiple Choice. Select the one best answer for each question.

53. To find information about care to be given to an individual patient, you should consult the

    a. patient's medical chart.   c. patient care plan.

    b. procedure manual.   d. nursing policy manual.

54. For the most up-to-date information about the patient's condition, check the:

    a. patient's medical chart.   c. procedure manual.

    b. nursing policy manual.   d. patient's care plan.

55. The patient's chart:

    a. is not a permanent document.

    b. is a legal document.

    c. is properly written in pencil.

    d. may be used only while the patient is in the hospital facility.

56. When reporting off duty, your report should include:

    a. details on how your day went.

    b. the care you gave each patient.

    c. comments about patients not in your care.

    d. observations of how well the staff got along.

57. Nursing assistants may document on the:

    a. physician's order sheet.   c. dietary record.

    b. consultant record.   d. flow sheet.

58. Charting must

    a. be about all the patients in one room.

    b. address problems listed in the patient's care plan.

    c. include the wishes of the family.

    d. none of these.

59. When charting,

    a. use objective statements.

    b. use complete sentences.

    c. make up abbreviations to save space.

    d. round off times to the closest hour.

60. Your patient has a kidney condition. You should note

    a. rate of respirations.   c. vaginal drainage.

    b. edema   d. appetite

61. Your patient has a digestive problem. You should note

    a. color of sputum.

    b. orientation to time.

    c. belching.

    d. lumps.

62. Your patient has a heart problem. you should note

    a. regularity of pulse.

    b. mental status.

    c. nasal drainage.

    d. ability to walk.

Matching. Match the regular time and its equivalent in international time.

Regular Time	International Time	
63. _____ 12:30 AM	a. 1230	e. 2000
64. _____ 7:15 AM	b. 1915	f. 0030
65. _____ 2:30 PM	c. 0800	g. 0715
66. _____ 8 PM	d. 1430	h. 1630
67. _____ 4:30 PM		

Completion. Complete each statement as it relates to the charting by selecting the proper word from those provided.

blank	clearly	color	completely	entry
error	patient	sequence	spell	title

68. Fill out new headings _____ .

69. Use correct _____ of ink.

70. Date and time each _____ .

71. Chart entries in correct _____ .

72. Print or write _____ .

73. _____ each word correctly.

74. Leave no _____ spaces between entries.

75. Do not use the word _____ .

76. Sign each entry with first initial, last name, and _____ .

77. Make correction by drawing one line through entry and print the word _____ on the line with your initials.

Clinical Situations. Answer the following questions in regard to this patient's care.

Robert Gonzales is 62 years of age. He is post brain attack. He shows right side weakness, alteration in cerebral tissue perfusion, and aphasia. The nurse has instructed you to assist with all ADLs. The patient showers. Vital signs are to be checked T.I.D.

78. How many times each day will you measure the patient's vital signs?

_____

79. What kind of help might this patient need in ADLs?

_____

80. What particular safety measure must you take during the shower?

_____

81. What problem must be handled due to the aphasia?

_____

82. Explain the meanings of the following conditions.

    a. right side weakness _____

    _____

    b. alteration in cerebral tissue perfusion _____

    _____

    c. Will raising your voice help Mr. Gonzales understand?

    _____

    _____

    d. What are two nonverbal communication techniques that speech therapists sometimes use to help a patient with aphasia?

    _____

    _____

DEVELOPING GREATER INSIGHT

83. Examine some unidentified care plans. Try giving an oral report based on the information.
84. Select a partner. Using your senses to make observations, describe the signs or symptoms you identify.

UNIT 9   Meeting Basic Human Needs

OBJECTIVES

As a result of this unit, you will be able to:
- Spell and define terms.
- Describe the stages of human growth and development.
- List five physical needs of patients.
- List four reasons why patients have difficulty sleeping.
- Define self-esteem.
- Describe how the nursing assistant can meet the patient's emotional needs.
- Discuss methods of dealing with the fearful patient.
- List nursing assistant actions to ensure that patients have the opportunity for intimacy.
- List the guidelines to assist patients in meeting their spiritual needs.

UNIT SUMMARY

Individuals develop at varying rates. There are, however, some well-defined developmental stages through which each person passes.
- Certain developmental skills are characteristically acquired at certain stages of life—from birth to death. A person's success in mastering these skills affects the progress of his development.
- Regardless of developmental level, people have common basic emotional and physical needs.
- The nursing staff must be sensitive to the influence of culture on the expression of individual needs.
- The way these needs are expressed varies, especially when a person is ill.
- The nursing staff must be sensitive to these individual needs. They must find ways of successfully providing for them.

NURSING ASSISTANT ALERT

Action	Benefit
Recognize that age groups differ in levels of development	Each patient will be treated as an individual.
Accept people as unique individuals with basic needs.	Care plans will be developed that consider and meet personal needs.

ACTIVITIES

Vocabulary Exercise. Unscramble the words introduced in this unit and define them. Select terms from the list provided.

commodes	growth	preadolescence	development
intimacy	urinal	feces	orthopneic

1. C E I O T R N H O P _____

2. C E C A E N R E L D O P E S _____

3. A R L I N U _____

4. W G O R H T _____

5. P O N L E E V D T E M _____

6. T I M A C I N Y _____

7. C F E E S _____

8. M E S O D M C O _____

Matching.

9. In the play room for ambulatory patients you find six children to check. Indicate which is demonstrating appropriate behavior for his or her age group.

   Behavior = a. appropriate or b. inappropriate

   a. _____ Scott 16, is receiving an IV and is talking to Patty, 17, who is 2 days postoperative following an appendectomy.

   b. _____ Bobbi, age 10, is sitting alone stringing large beads.

   c. _____ Felicia, age 8, and Kimmie, 11, are playing parchesi.

   d. _____ Tommy, 4, and Brian, 5, are playing with the wooden cars and trucks.

   e. _____ Jonnie, 2½, is playing with blocks near the older boys.

   f. _____ Dona, age 3, is sitting near Jonnie, pushing different shaped blocks through different shaped holes in the cover of a box.

10. Match the proper term on the right with the explanation of sexual expression on the left.

    a. _____ sexual attraction to members of both sexes   1. masturbation

    b. _____ self-stimulation for sexual pleasure   2. homosexuality

    c. _____ sexual attraction between members of the same sex   3. bisexuality

    d. _____ sexual attraction to members of opposite sex   4. heterosexuality

Completion. Complete the statements in the spaces provided.

11. The stages of growth and development refer to the _____ that must be mastered before moving on to the next stage.

12. Jimmy Hinkle is 12 months old. He weighs 16 pounds and is 26 inches tall. You know this is _____ than average for his chronological age.

13. The average vocabulary of a two-year-old is about _____ words.

14. Five characteristics of early adulthood include:

   a. _____

   b. _____

   c. _____

   d. _____

   e. _____

15. The sandwich generation of middle age refers to _____

_____

16. Later maturity is characterized by a period of _____

Brief Answers.   Briefly answer the following questions or directions.

17. Explain Erickson's belief regarding personality development.

_____

_____

18. Briefly explain Maslow's theory regarding human needs.

_____

_____

_____

19. List five general points to keep in mind when assisting patients to meet their nutritional needs.

   a. _____

   b. _____

   c. _____

   d. _____

   e. _____

Clinical Situations.   Briefly explain why you think the patient is reacting this way and how you think the nursing assistant should react to the following situations.

20. Jeannie Hunt, 16, has been diagnosed as suffering from osteosarcoma of her right tibia. The prognosis is guarded and she has been scheduled for surgery to remove the right leg at mid-calf, to be followed by radiation. She asks to see the youth leader of her church.

_____

_____

21. Craig Martin, 52, is recovering from a partial prostatectomy. He is complaining loudly about his care, the food, and the other patients in the room.

_____

_____

22. Lucy Sneider, 26, is having difficulty sleeping at bedtime. She is in your care.

_____

_____

23. You are serving nourishments and find the door to Rudolph Baker's room closed.

_____

24. You are assigned to care for the two male patients in Room 762. You have reason to believe that they may be lovers and another nursing assistant asks you what you know about their relationship.

   _____

25. Every time you enter Belinda Mitchell's room, she tries to make sexual advances to you and to find reasons to touch you.

   _____

RELATING TO THE NURSING PROCESS

Write the step of the nursing process that is related to the nursing assistant action.

Nursing Assistant Action   **Nursing Process Step**

26. The nursing assistant assists the mature adult to ambulate.   _____

27. The nursing assistant reports that the 18-month-old baby has difficulty sitting up.   _____

28. The nursing assistant reports that the teenager is still having periods of depression.   _____

29. The nursing assistant assists the patient with his oxygen.   _____

UNIT 10   Developing Cultural Sensitivity

OBJECTIVES

As a result of this unit, you will be able to:

- Spell and define terms.

- Name six major cultural groups in the United States.

- Describe ways the major cultures differ in their family organization, communication, need for personal space, health practices, religion, and traditions.

- List ways nursing assistants can develop sensitivity about cultures other than their own.

- State ways the nursing assistant can demonstrate appreciation of and sensitivity to other cultures.

- List ways the nursing assistant can help patients in practicing rituals appropriate to their cultures.

UNIT SUMMARY

Patients have a variety of cultural heritages. These heritages influence how individuals:

- Communicate.

- React to health concerns.

- View one another and the need for personal space.

- Celebrate holidays.

- Select foods.

- Practice religions beliefs.

Six ethnic groups predominate in the United States. They are:

- Caucasians.

- African Americans.

- Hispanics.

- Asian/Pacific.

- Native Americans.

- Middle Eastern/Arabs.

Nursing assistants must treat all patients as individuals and be sensitive to:

- The patient's acceptance of caregivers.

- The amount of disrobing permitted.

- The degree of touch that is comfortable.

NURSING ASSISTANT ALERT

Action	Benefit
Learn as much as possible about a patient's culture.	Helps patients receive more personalized care.
Treat patients as individuals within a culture.	Assures that care will be personalized.
Be sensitive to patients' needs relating to personal space, touching, and religious practices.	Increases patient's sense of acceptance and respect.

ACTIVITIES

Vocabulary Exercise. Complete the puzzle by filling in the missing letters. Use the definitions to help you discover the words.

```
                P
1.   _ _ _ _ E _ _ _ _ _ _
                R
2.   _ _ _ _ S _ _ _ _
                O
3.   _ _ _ N _ _ _ _ _
                A
4.   _ _ _ L _ _ _
5.   _ _ _ S _ _ _ _ _ _ _ _
                P
6.      _ A _ _
                C
7.   _ _ _ E _
```

Definitions

1. Beliefs that are rigid and based on generalizations.

2. Engraved objects used to ward off evil.

3. Special group within a race as defined by national origin/culture.

4. Charm against evil.

5. Ability to be aware of and to appreciate personal characteristics of others.

6. Classification of people according to shared physical characteristics.

7. Customs.

Brief Answers. Briefly answer the following questions.

8. What are the six major ethnic groups in the United States?

   a. _____

   b. _____

   c. _____

   d. _____

   e. _____

   f. _____

9. What is meant by "cross-cultural" nursing? _____

   _____

   _____

10. What effect does living in a new culture have on the cultural values and traditions of the country of origin?_____

_____

_____

11. People are classified as a race according to which shared physical characteristics? _____

_____

_____

_____

12. What features do members of ethnic groups share in common?

_____

_____

_____

_____

13. What are five cultural differences that exist between ethnic groups?

a. _____

b. _____

c. _____

d. _____

e. _____

14. What are three beliefs shared by members of a culture?

a. _____

b. _____

c. _____

15. What are the five major religions in the United States?

a. _____

b. _____

c. _____

d. _____

e. _____

True/False. Mark the following true or false by circling T or F.

16. T   F   Family organization determines who is responsible for health care.

17. T   F   In Caucasian families, the father is the dominant decision maker.

18. T   F   In extended families, caregiving and personal care are personal and shared responsibilities.

19. T   F   A nuclear family usually includes aunts, uncles, and grandparents.

20. T   F   African-Americans prefer to stand far away (more than 3 feet) when speaking to others.

21. T   F   Asians consider direct eye contact inappropriate.

22. T   F   Prolonged eye contact is considered disrespectful by Hispanics.

23. T   F   It is proper for only men to shake hands in Middle Eastern countries.

24. T   F   Uncovering the shoulders of a person from India may be considered disrespectful.

25. T   F   People who are bilingual revert to their language of origin when under stress.

26. T   F   Dialects may vary between different groups who share a common culture.

RELATING TO THE NURSING PROCESS

Write the step of the nursing process that is related to the nursing assistant action.

Nursing Assistant Action	Nursing Process Step
27. The nursing assistant reports her observations that the patient cannot speak and understand English easily.	_____
28. The nursing assistant stands at a distance that is comfortable for the patient when giving care.	_____
29. The nursing assistant asks politely about practices that are unfamiliar.	_____
30. The nursing assistant provides privacy when a spiritual advisor visits.	_____

DEVELOPING GREATER INSIGHT

31. Your patient, Mr. Dang, is 82 and has lived in this country for several years. He was born in Vietnam, is a Buddhist, and is bilingual.

    a. Of what major ethnic group is Mr. Dang a member?

    _____

    b. How might he view the cause of his illness?

    _____

    c. What responsibility do you think his family might feel toward his care?

    _____

    d. What diety would Mr. Dang worship?

    _____

    e. As a culture, how do Asian-Americans feel about direct eye contact?

    _____

    f. Why would it be unwise to stereotype this person?

    _____

32. Your patient, Ms. Ruiz, is 76. Her leg was fractured in several places when she was hit by a car. She is in balanced traction on your unit. She is originally from Costa Rica and speaks Spanish with limited English. She tells you that her "humors" are out of balance and that she is being punished for past sins. She wants to see a curandera.

    a. How might you improve your ability to communicate with her?

    _____

    b. What four religious articles might be important to her?

    _____

    c. In what religious ceremony might she wish to participate?

    _____

    d. What are the four humors to which she refers?

    _____

UNIT 11   Infection

OBJECTIVES

As a result of this unit, you will be able to:

- Spell and define terms.
- Identify the most common microbes and describe some of their characteristics.
- Define infectious disease.
- Name five serious infectious diseases.
- Identify the causes of several important infectious diseases.
- List the ways that infectious diseases are spread.
- List the steps of the chain of infection.
- Describe common treatments for infectious disease.
- List natural body defenses against infections.
- Explain why patients are at risk for infections.

UNIT SUMMARY

Pathogens are microscopic organisms that cause disease. Pathogens differ from one another in the way they:

- Look.
- Cause disease.
- Grow.

Pathogens:

- Enter and leave the body by special routes known as portals of entry and exit.
- Transmit disease by direct and indirect means.
- May be kept alive in reservoirs.

Major types of pathogens include:

- Bacteria.
- Fungi.
- Protozoa.

Protection against infectious disease may be achieved with:

- Natural defenses.
- Artificial techniques.

Immunization by vaccine to form antibodies against certain infectious diseases is an important form of protection.

NURSING ASSISTANT ALERT

Action	Benefit
Learn the names and characteristics of common microbes.	Achieve better understanding of the nature of germs, transmission, and control.
Relate the infection process to the transmission of infection.	Achieve control over disease transmission. Ensures safety of patients and health care providers.
Take appropriate immunizations.	Protects patients and health care providers from infection.

ACTIVITIES

Vocabulary Exercise. Complete the crossword puzzle by using the definitions presented.

Down

1. Artificial or weakened antigen
2. Rod-shaped microbes
3. Contaminated objects
4. Organisms that cause disease

Across

5. Drugs used to control infection
6. Poisons produced by microbes
7. One who harbors organisms
8. Community of organisms
9. A person who harbors and transmits infectious disease without being ill himself
10. Inflammation of the liver
11. Single-celled form of fungus

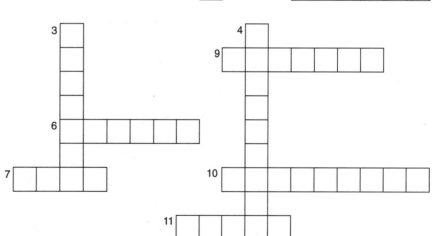
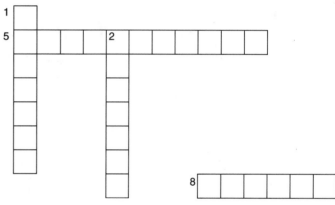

Matching. Match the term and the description.

Description   Term

12. _____ round bacterium growing in chains   a. antigen

13. _____ simple one-celled organisms that cause malaria   b. bacilli

14. _____ pathogenic microbe that stimulates the   c. contagious
            production of antibodies   d. streptococci

15. _____ systemic bacterial infection spread through the bloodstream e. vector

16. _____ capable of passing the infection to others   f. parasite

17. _____ spitting up blood   g. protozoa

18. _____ organism that grows best on living matter   h. hemoptysis

19. _____ rod-shaped microbes   i. staphylococci

20. _____ microbes that grow in pairs   j. bacteremia

21. _____ microbes that grow in clusters   k. diplococci

Match the type of organism and the diseases commonly caused.

Disease   Organism

22. _____ diarrhea   a. bacterium

23. _____ abscess   b. virus

24. _____ vulvovaginitis   c. protozoan

25. _____ inflammation of the brain   d. yeast

26. _____ herpes   e. mold

27. _____ hepatitis

28. _____ boil

29. _____ common cold

30. _____ toxic shock

31. _____ athlete's foot

Completion. Complete the statements in the spaces provided.

32. List four external mechanisms against disease.

    a. _____

    b. _____

    c. _____

    d. _____

33. List four internal defense mechanisms against disease.

    a. _____

    b. _____

    c. _____

    d. _____

34. A human carrier is a person who _____

    _____

35. List the five major portals of entry.

    a. _____

    b. _____

    c. _____

    d. _____

    e. _____

36. List seven portals of exit.

    a. _____

    b. _____

    c. _____

    d. _____

    e. _____

    f. _____

    g. _____

37. The causative agent of infectious disease means the _____

    _____

38. In the health care setting, three potential reservoirs of infection must be considered and controlled. They are:

    a. _____

    b. _____

    c. _____

39. List three ways microbes may be spread.

    a. _____

    b. _____

    c. _____

40. Name the six components of the chain of infection.

    a. _____

    b. _____

    c. _____

    d. _____

    e. _____

    f. _____

41. List five signs and symptoms of influenza.

    a. _____

    b. _____

    c. _____

    d. _____

    e. _____

42. Three common viruses that cause hepatitis are:

    a. _____

    b. _____

    c. _____

43. Two groups of organisms that have become resistant to methicillin and vancomycin are:

    a. methicillin-resistant _____

    b. vancomycin-resistant _____

True/False. Mark the following true or false by circling T or F.

44. T   F   People who are HIV-positive are less resistant to tuberculosis.

45. T   F   The barrier that forms around the tuberculosis infection is called an abscess.

46. T   F   Weight gain is a sign associated with tuberculosis infection.

47. T   F   A positive Mantoux test indicates the presence of antibodies to tuberculosis.

Clinical Situations.

48. Alan Corbin, 19 years old, is in end-stage AIDS. He is your patient. Mark the following questions true or false to demonstrate your understanding of the disease.

    a. T   F   The disease is caused by a bacterium.

    b. T   F   Everyone who comes in contact with the organism becomes ill with AIDS.

    c. T   F   An asymptomatic period may last from months to years following infection.

    d. T   F   Progression of the disease process is determined by the effect of the viruses on the red blood cells.

    e. T   F   Flulike symptoms, night sweats, and swollen lymph nodes are some of the early symptoms.

    f. T   F   Tests are available to measure the level of viral activity in a patient's blood.

    g. T   F   Protease inhibitors can cure the disease.

    h. T   F   There is no evidence that touching or hugging an AIDS patient will transmit the disease.

49. Amy Lee, 87, was admitted to your unit. Her admission diagnosis was lobar pneumonia. Her initial vital signs included T 104.4°F P 112 R 24 (labored). She is 5'6" and weighs 89 pounds. She is generally in poor health, presenting a history of emphysema and congestive heart failure. What factors do you believe might have contributed to her current health state?

    a. _____

    b. _____

    c. _____

50. Mrs. Bustemonte is 67 years of age and a patient on your unit. She has an indwelling catheter. She has a urinary tract infection and urinates frequently. She tells you that she has burning on urination. She also has an elevated temperature (100.8°F). List four actions you should take when caring for her. Choose terms from the list provided.

    adequate   back   catheter   empty

    front   less   urine

    a. Assist in maintaining _____ fluid levels.

    b. Report to the nurse if she eats _____ food.

    c. Assist with toileting to keep the bladder _____ .

d. Clean the perineal area wiping from _____ to _____ .

e. Perform _____ care as directed.

f. Report changes in the character of the _____ .

51. Complete the chain of infection.

a. _____

b. _____

c. _____

d. _____

RELATING TO THE NURSING PROCESS

Nursing Assistant Action	Nursing Process Step
52. The nursing assistant reports an elevation of Mr. Bergen's temperature and redness near his infusion site.	_____
53. The nursing assistant makes sure Mr. Popejoy, who has pneumonia, has plenty of tissues and a place to dispose of them.	_____
54. The nursing assistant reports that Mr. Menendez is coughing frequently as he is admitted.	_____

DEVELOPING GREATER INSIGHT

55. _____ Receiving antibiotics when infected.

56. _____ Disinfecting bedpans.

57. _____ Covering a draining bedsore.

58. _____ Not coming to work when you have a cold.

59. _____ Putting a Band-aid® on a cut in your skin.

a. protecting the portal of entry

b. protecting the portal of exit

c. protecting susceptible host

d. controlling the causative agents

e. eliminating the reservoir

60. Discuss with the class the value of immunization procedures. Try to answer the following:

a. Which vaccines are commonly given?

b. When should vaccines be given?

c. How do vaccines offer protection?

d. Are there some infections for which there are no immunizations?

e. How can you protect yourself against infections for which there is no immunization?

UNIT 12   Infection Control

OBJECTIVES

As a result of this unit, you will be able to:

- Define and spell all vocabulary words and terms.
- Explain the principles of medical asepsis.
- Explain the components of standard precautions.
- List the types of personal protective equipment.
- Describe nursing assistant actions related to standard precautions.
- Describe airborne precautions.
- Describe droplet precautions.
- Describe contact precautions.
- Demonstrate the following:

Procedure 1	Handwashing
Procedure 2	Putting on a Mask
Procedure 3	Putting on a Gown
Procedure 4	Putting on Gloves
Procedure 5	Removing Contaminated Gloves
Procedure 6	Removing Contaminated Gloves, Mask, and Gown
Procedure 7	Serving a Meal in an Isolation Unit
Procedure 8	Measuring Vital Signs in an Isolation Unit
Procedure 9	Transferring Nondisposable Equipment Outside of Isolation Unit
Procedure 10	Specimen Collection from Patient in an Isolation Unit
Procedure 11	Caring for Linens in an Isolation Unit
Procedure 12	Transporting Patient to and from Isolation Unit
Procedure 13	Opening a Sterile Package

UNIT SUMMARY

When patients have communicable diseases that are easily transmitted to others, special techniques must be used. The patient is placed in isolation. Everyone coming into contact with the patient must practice appropriate isolation techniques. The emphasis is on the infectious material that carries the specific microorganisms. The goal of the health care provider is to interrupt the chain of infection by preventing the transmission of the microbes. By working toward this goal, the health care provider protects the patient, the environment, and self.

The spread of disease can be controlled by:

- Conscientious handwashing.
- Proper medical and surgical asepsis.
- Understanding and faithfully following:

  Standard precautions.
  Transmission-based precautions.
  Isolation techniques.
  Disinfection and sterilization procedures.

NURSING ASSISTANT ALERT

Action	Benefit
Follow standard precautions exactly.	Prevents transfer of infectious materials.
Give extra attention to isolation patients.	Prevents patient from feeling abandoned.
Place sharps in proper container.	Decreases the danger of needle or sharp sticks.
Follow specific transmission-based precautions as outlined in care plan.	Eliminates unnecessary actions while ensuring specific transmission prevention techniques.
Follow aseptic techniques carefully and accurately.	Protects patients and health care providers from infection.

ACTIVITIES

Vocabulary Exercise. Put a circle around the word defined. Use the terms in the list provided.

CDC	communicable	dirty	disposable	droplet
Feces	gloves	goggles	gown	HEPA
HIV	isolate	negative	standard	universe

```
S Q D I S O L A T E L E
S L A I T W B Y C R L M
N E S P S K P P L B C T
O V E G E P J X A D Y C
I I L E N H O C C L M A
T T G N Q J I S N M E T
E A G A U N S H A T F N
R G O H U P W W L B T O
C E G M D I R T Y V L C
X N M A (D) R O P L E T E
E O H S T A N D A R D N
C S E F E C E S G O W N
```

1. spread long distances in the air on dust and moisture
2. Centers for Disease Control and Prevention
3. an infectious disease easily transmitted to others
4. protective hand coverings
5. expendable
6. separating ill patients from others
7. waste products of the body
8. eye protection that is always worn with a mask
9. one type of mask used in airborne precautions
10. human immunodeficiency virus
11. air flow in an airborne precautions room is reversed creating a _____ pressure environment
12. unclean
13. _____ precautions are used any time contact with blood, body fluid, secretions, excretions, mucous membranes, or nonintact skin is likely
14. PPE that covers the uniform

True/False. Mark the following true or false by circling T or F.

15. T   F   Linen found on a linen cart is considered clean.

16. T   F   Linen that has touched the floor is clean as long as the floor is not wet.

17. T   F   Medical aseptic techniques destroy all organisms on an article.

18. T   F   One patient's articles may be used by another as long as the first patient doesn't have a communicable disease.

When washing hands correctly

19. T   F   Always use cool water.

20. T   F   Lean against the sink so no water will get on the floor.

21. T   F   A soap dispenser is preferable to a bar of soap.

22. T   F   Always rinse the bar of soap (if used) after use.

23. T   F   Turn faucets on and off with gloves.

24. T   F   Always point fingertips up when washing.

25. T   F   It is the use of soap that actually removes microbes from hands.

26. T   F   Hands can be washed effectively in 10 to 15 seconds.

27. T   F   Personal medical asepsis includes a daily bath.

28. T   F   Complete personal protective equipment is required when working with all patients.

Completion. Complete the statements in the spaces provided.

29. The purpose of transmission-based precautions is _____

30. When working in droplet precautions, a mask is worn when you work within _____ feet of the patient.

31. Isolation is the responsibility of _____

32. The purpose of wearing a mask and gown in the isolation unit is to _____

33. Gloves should be used whenever there may be contact with _____

34. To be effective, a mask must cover both _____

35. A gown should only be used _____

36 The contaminated gown should be folded _____ before disposing of it in the proper receptacle.

37. Disposable equipment is used only _____

38. List seven secretions or excretions that are potentially infectious.

    a. _____   e. _____

    b. _____   f. _____

    c. _____   g. _____

    d. _____

39. Breaks in the skin of a health care worker should be immediately treated by _____ and applying

    _____.

40. What do these six items have in common before they are used?

stethoscope	glass thermometer	bathtub
shower chair	tympanic thermometer	wheelchair

Brief Answers.

41. State the name applied to the type of infection control that is used with all situations in which care providers may contact body fluids._____

42. List the three types of transmission-based precautions.

    a. _____

    b. _____

    c. _____

43. List three ways communicable diseases may be spread.

    a. _____

    b. _____

    c. _____

44. List six articles to be placed on a cart outside an isolation room.

    a. _____   d. _____

    b. _____   e. _____

    c. _____   f. _____

45. State the sequence for applying personal protective equipment.

    a. _____

    b. _____

    c. _____

    d. _____

    e. _____

46. List seven precautions to keep in mind when handling soiled linen.

    a. _____

    b. _____

    c. _____

    d. _____

    e. _____

    f. _____

    g. _____

47. State the measures that are to be taken to care for vital sign equipment used with the patient in isolation.

    a. _____

    b. _____

48. Explain the care of food not eaten by a patient in isolation.

_____

49. Name the type of bag that is used for the transport of specimens.

_____

50. Name two ways to sterilize an item.

    a. _____

    b. _____

Clinical Situations. Briefly describe how a nursing assistant should react to the following situations.

51. You saw an airborne precautions sign on Mr. Keene's door. You are assigned to serve his breakfast tray. _____

_____

_____

52. You are responsible for caring for nondisposable equipment from a contact precautions unit.

_____

Identification.

53. Identify the sign and indicate the type of precaution to be used.

a. _____

_____

_____

_____

_____

b. _____

_____

_____

_____

_____

c. _____

_____

_____

_____

_____

d. _____

_____

_____

_____

_____

e. _____

_____

_____

_____

_____

54. Identify what is wrong with this picture. What should be done to correct it? Please show two nursing assistants.

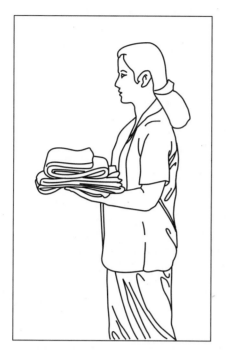
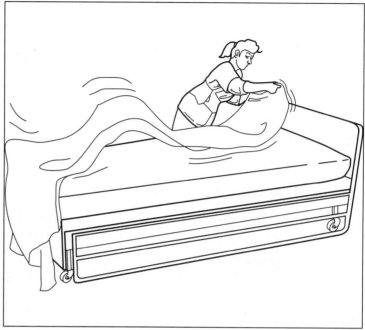

a. Error _____   c. Error _____

b. Correction _____   d. Correction _____

55. What is wrong with the figure on the left? Correct it in the figure on the right.

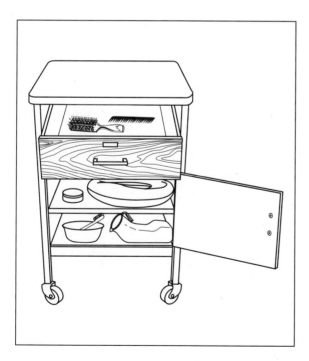
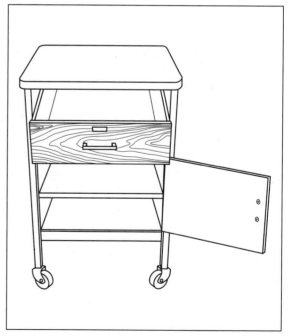

a. Error _____

b. Correction _____

Use the empty bedside table to demonstrate the correction by locating the articles properly or writing in the words.

56. Briefly explain how the nursing assistant should react to the following. You are assisting the nurse in setting up a sterile field to change a surgical dressing. You open some 4 x 4's and reach across the field and place them on the towel. The nurse tells you the setup cannot be used and must be done again. Why?

_____

_____

RELATING TO THE NURSING PROCESS

Write the step of the nursing process that is related to the nursing assistant action.

Nursing Assistant Action   **Nursing Process Step**

57. The nursing assistant isn't sure about how to transport the patient safely from isolation to the x-ray department so she asks the team leader for instructions.   _____

58. The nursing assistant carefully removes the contaminated gown and disposes of it properly after completing care in the contact precautions room.   _____

DEVELOPING GREATER INSIGHT

59. With classmates and teacher, explain ways to help patients feel less abandoned when in isolation.

60. Investigate the transmission-based isolation precautions in your facility and report back to the class.

61. Discuss why direct contact with blood and body fluids can be dangerous to a health care worker.

UNIT 13   Environmental and Nursing Assistant Safety

OBJECTIVES

As a result of this unit, you will be able to:

- Spell and define terms.
- Describe the health care facility environment.
- Identify measures to promote environmental safety.
- List situations when equipment must be repaired.
- Describe the elements required for fire.
- List five measures to prevent fire.
- Describe the procedure to follow if fire occurs.
- Demonstrate the use of a fire extinguisher.
- List techniques for using ergonomics on the job.
- Demonstrate appropriate body mechanics.
- Describe the types of information contained in Material Safety Data Sheets (MSDS).

UNIT SUMMARY

The nursing staff is responsible for maintaining a safe, comfortable environment for the patient.

- The bed and unit are the patient's home during the hospital stay.
- All equipment must be readily available and kept in clean operating condition.
- Safety is the business of everyone. Knowing the rules ensures your full participation.
- The cleanliness of the unit must be maintained on a daily basis. The unit must be completely cleaned before being used by a new patient.
- Fire is a potential threat. All staff must be aware of the factors that contribute to fire hazard and control them. Fire plans must be understood and followed in case of a fire.
- Knowledge of ergonomics can prevent worker injuries.
- Knowledge of chemicals used is required by federal law.

NURSING ASSISTANT ALERT

Action	Benefit
Maintain an even temperature, regulating light and ventilation.	Contributes to patient comfort.
Report equipment in need of repair.	Prevents possible accidents and injury.

Action	Benefit
Use proper body mechanics.	Avoids injury to patient and caregiver.
Apply restraints and supports according to established protocol.	Ensures proper standard of patient care.
Know and follow fire safety policies.	Ensures patient and staff greatest opportunities for safe exit during a fire emergency.

ACTIVITIES

Vocabulary Exercise. Each line has four different spellings of a word from this unit. Circle the correctly spelled word.

1. incident	incedent	incidant	incydent
2. ralys	rails	riles	rhales
3. warde	werd	ward	whard
4. privite	privat	pryvate	private
5. ergonomecs	ergonomics	erkonomics	ergonomicks
6. concurent	concurrent	concurrant	concarrent
7. seme private	semiprivote	semepryvate	semiprivate
8. envyromental	environmantyl	environmental	enviromental

Completion. Complete the statements related to safety practices in the spaces provided by selecting the correct term from the list provided.

alcohol	all health care	available to the patient	calm
checked	concern	electrical	fuel
grounded	hazard	heat	incident
indirect	locked	MSDS	nail polish
never	oils	OSHA	oxygen
patients	right away	screens, curtains	shut off
supervisor	tagged	upright	work
work related	70	your bare hands	

9. Keeping the environment safe and clean is the responsibility of _____ workers.

10. Prevention of injuries to patients and others is of primary _____ .

11. Wheels should always be _____ unless a bed is being moved.

12. The best temperature for the patient's room is about _____ degrees.

13. The best way to shield patients from drafts is by _____ or _____ .

14. The best kind of light is _____ .

15. When leaving the patient's room, be sure that the ceiling lights are _____ .

16. Frayed _____ cords should be reported at once.

17. For safety, never pick up broken glass with _____ .

18. An accident that occurs in a health care facility is called an _____ .

19. When equipment is broken, it is _____ .

20. Mechanical lifts should be _____ before use.

21. Plugs that are not properly _____ are a fire hazard.

22. Smoking in bed should _____ be permitted.

23. Make sure signal lights are always _____ .

24. The three elements that form the fire triangle are _____, _____, and _____ .

25. Possible fire hazards should be reported _____ to the _____ .

26. When oxygen is in use, flammable liquids such as _____, _____, or _____ should not be used.

27. A fire extinguisher should be carried in the _____ position.

28. When there is an emergency, it is very important for you to keep _____ .

29. When there is a fire, always move _____ to safety first.

30. The term ergonomic means _____ .

31. The federal agency that is responsible for employees' safety is called _____ .

32. Hazard communication called _____ must be supplied by manufacturers by law.

Brief Answers. Write the information in the spaces provided.

33. Briefly list nine components included in the patient's environment.

  a. _____   f. _____

  b. _____   g. _____

  c. _____   h. _____

  d. _____   i. _____

  e. _____

34. Name two pieces of fire control equipment.

  a. _____   b. _____

35. The acronym PASS is important for fire control. The:

  a. P stands for _____

  b. A stands for _____

  c. S stands for _____

  d. S stands for _____

36. List six ergonomic techniques you can use to decrease the risk of an incident.

  a. _____

  b. _____

  c. _____

  d. _____

  e. _____

  f. _____

37. State three types of information you expect to learn from the MSDS of a product.

  a. _____

  b. _____

  c. _____

38. Draw the fire triangle, showing its elements.

Hidden Picture. Look carefully at the picture and list each violation of a safety measure in the space provided.

39. _____

40. _____

41. _____

42. _____

43. _____

44. _____

45. _____

46. _____

47. _____

48. _____

49. _____

50. _____

51. _____

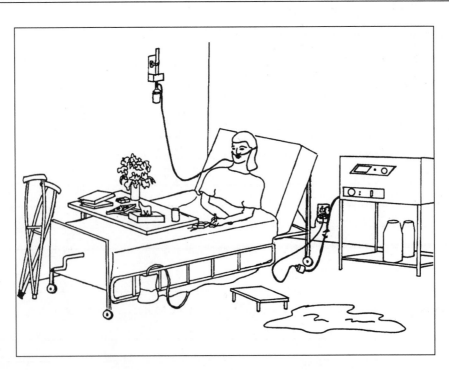

RELATING TO THE NURSING PROCESS

Write the step of the nursing process that is related to the nursing assistant action.

Nursing Assistant Action	Nursing Process Step
52. The nursing assistant participates in a conference regarding patient evacuation in case of an emergency.	_____
53. The nursing team, including the nursing assistants, takes part in a training session to prepare for actions during a patient arrest.	_____

DEVELOPING GREATER INSIGHT

54. Discuss with classmates why consistent attention to safety helps to create feelings of security for the patient when in the hospital.

55. Investigate the location of escape routes for your facility.

56. Practice with your instructor and classmates the proper way to operate fire control equipment.

UNIT 14   Patient Safety and Positioning

OBJECTIVES

As a result of this unit, you will be able to:

- Spell and define terms.

- List the elements that are common to all procedures.

- Identify patients who are at risk for having incidents.

- List alternatives to the use of physical restraints.

- Describe the guidelines for the use of restraints.

- Demonstrate the correct application of restraints.

- Describe two measures for preventing these types of incidents: accidental poisoning, thermal injuries, skin injuries, and choking.

- Describe correct body alignment for the patient.

- List the purposes of repositioning patients.

- Demonstrate these positions using the correct supportive devices: supine, semisupine, prone, semiprone, lateral, Fowler's and orthopneic.

  Procedure 14 Turning the Patient Toward You
  Procedure 15 Turning the Patient Away from You
  Procedure 16 Moving a Patient to the Head of the Bed
  Procedure 17 Logrolling the Patient

UNIT SUMMARY

- Preventive measures must be implemented to avoid patient incidents.

- Restraints, if necessary, must be applied correctly and all policies followed.

- Care must be taken to keep the patient in good alignment and provide support at all times in all positions.

- Frequent change of position helps prevent deformities and decubiti. It also aids general body functions and contributes to comfort.

- Frequent position changes are essential to prevent:

  Musculoskeletal deformities and loss of calcium from bone.
  Poor skin nutrition and the development of pressure sores.
  Respiratory complications such as pneumonia.
  Decreased circulation that could lead to thrombophlebitis and renal calculi.
  Loss of opportunities for social exchange between patient and staff.

- Procedures are step-by-step directions for giving patient care. They must be followed faithfully.

- Some steps are common to all procedures. The beginning procedure actions and procedure completion actions include the following.

BEGINNING PROCEDURE ACTIONS

1. Wash your hands thoroughly.
2. Assemble equipment.
3. At the patient's room, knock and pause before entering the room.
4. Introduce yourself and identify the patient by checking his or her identification bracelet.
5. Ask visitors to leave the room and inform them where they may wait.
6. Provide privacy.
7. Explain what will happen and answer questions.
8. Allow the patient to assist as much as possible.
9. Raise the bed to a comfortable working height.
10. Carry out precautions gowning and gloving.
11. Use standard precautions when contact with blood, body fluids, mucous membranes, or nonintact skin is likely.

PROCEDURE COMPLETION ACTIONS

1. Position the patient comfortably.
2. Return the bed to the lowest horizontal position.
3. Leave signal cord, telephone, and fresh water where the patient can reach them.
4. Perform a general safety check of the patient and the environment.
5. Open privacy curtains.
6. Remove and discard personal protective equipment, if used, according to facility policy.
7. Care for equipment following facility policy.
8. Wash your hands.
9. Let visitors know when they may reenter the room.
10. Report completion of the task.
11. Document action and your observations.

NOTE: Where there are open lesions, wet linen, or possible contact with patient body fluids, blood, mucous membranes, or nonintact skin, disposable gloves are to be worn during the procedure. Put on gloves before contact with the patient or linen. Dispose of gloves according to facility policy after they are removed. **ALWAYS APPLY STANDARD PRECAUTIONS.**

■ Special procedures in this unit relate to positioning, supporting, and restraining patients in a safe, appropriate manner, using proper body mechanics.

NURSING ASSISTANT ALERT

Action	Benefit
Assume proper posture during all activities.	Allows the body to function at its best.

Action	Benefit
Follow the eight basic rules for effective body use.	Prevents injury and reduces fatigue
Support patients in proper alignment in all positions.	Improves comfort and relieves strain. Prevents deformities. Allows body to function more effectively.
Apply restraints and supports according to established protocol.	Ensures proper standard of patient care.

ACTIVITIES

Vocabulary Exercise. Complete the puzzle by filling in the missing letters of words found in this unit. Use the definitions to help you discover these words.

1.   __ P __ __ __ __   1. Involving muscle contractions
2.   __ __ __ __ O __ __ __   2. Devices for maintaining the position of extremities
3.   __ __ S __ __ __ __ __ __   3. Device that inhibits patient movement
4.   __ __ __ __ __ I __ __   4. Ability to move
5.   __ __ __ T __ __ __ __ __ __ __   5. Occurs when muscles become fixed in one position
6.   __ __ __ I __ __   6. On the back
7.   __ __ O __ __ __ __ __ __   7. Steps to follow to carry out a task
8.   __ __ __ __ N __   8. Another term for orthosis

Completion. Complete the statements in the spaces provided.

9. Before beginning any patient contact, you must _____, _____ the patient, and, if appropriate, _____ .

10. A good principle to follow is never to attempt _____ to lift or move a patient who weighs more than you do.

11. A heavy or helpless patient can be more easily moved if a _____ is used.

12. A good way to help a patient maintain a side-lying position is to form a pillow roll and place it _____ _____

13. Before rolling a patient away from you, be sure the _____ _____

14. When moving the patient to the head of the bed, the nursing assistant should _____ the foot of the bed.

15. The position of a patient must be changed at least every _____ .

16. In the prone position, the bed is in the _____ position and the patient is placed on his _____ .

17. Two forms of restraint are _____ and _____ .

18. When restraints are released, the patient must be _____ .

19. Three incidents that may occur are _____ , _____ , and _____ injury.

True/False. Mark the following true or false by circling T or F.

20. T F Restraints should be used only as a last resort.

21. T F Side rails may safely be left down when restraints are in use.

22. T F Restraints should be secured to the immovable part of the bed frame.

23. T F To prevent accidental poisoning, store a patient's personal food items in the bedside table.

24. T F When preparing bath water, always turn the hot water on last.

25. T F Using a microwave oven to reheat foods is a safe, economical way because food is evenly heated.

26. T F Always knock before entering a room.

27. T F Special boots or shoes may be worn in bed to maintain feet in the proper alignment.

28. T F A patient positioned on his left side should be moved to the left side of the bed.

29. T F A trochanter roll should extend from under the arm, along the trunk, to the top of the hip.

Brief Answer. Briefly explain the reasoning behind each of the following statements.

30. The nursing assistant should use leg muscles and shoulder muscles to lift and not the muscles of the back. Why?

_____

31. Proper positioning of the patient's body must be conscientiously done because:

_____

_____

_____

32. The staff must take specific steps before applying restraints. What are the steps and why must they be done?

_____

_____

Name the Position. In the space provided on the left, name the position pictured on the right.

33. _____

34. _____

35. _____

Clinical Situations.

36. Mrs. Grover wears a hearing aid and glasses. She has difficulty ambulating and is unsteady on her feet. She is sometimes disoriented and tends to wander when she becomes hungry, in search of food. List ways a nursing assistant might protect this patient and avoid the need for protective restraints.

   a. _____

   b. _____

   c. _____

   d. _____

   e. _____

   f. _____

37. What physical restraints might be used if alternatives fail and the protocol for restraints has been followed?

   a. _____

   b. _____

   c. _____

   d. _____

   e. _____

38. Mr. Kinsey is 82 years of age, weighs 215 pounds, and has a respiratory problem (emphysema). He tends to slide to the foot of the bed and has difficulty being comfortable. What action should you take when you find him in this position?

   a. _____

   b. _____

   c. _____

39. Mr. Milhouse is 91 years of age and has difficulty swallowing since his brain attack. His left side is paralyzed and he needs assistance feeding himself. What might the nursing assistant do to help avoid aspiration?

   a. _____

   b. _____

   c. _____

   d. _____

   e. _____

   f. _____

   g. _____

   h. _____

DEVELOPING GREATER INSIGHT

40. Divide class into groups of two or three. With one person acting as the patient, have classmates practice positioning the patient using proper supports.

41. With classmates, practice applying restraints on one another, leaving them in place for 15 minutes. Think how you would feel if you wanted a drink of water or had to use the bathroom and no one was nearby to help you.

42. With classmates, practice positioning each other in the basic patient positions.

UNIT 15 The Patient's Mobility: Transfer Skills

OBJECTIVES

As a result of this unit, you will be able to:
- Spell and define terms.
- List the guidelines for safe transfers.
- Describe the difference between a standing transfer and a sitting transfer.
- Demonstrate correct application of a transfer belt.
- Demonstrate the following procedures:

  Procedure 18 Applying a Transfer Belt
  Procedure 19 Transferring the Patient from Bed to Chair—One Assistant
  Procedure 20 Transferring the Patient from Bed to Chair—Two Assistants
  Procedure 21 Transferring the Patient from Chair to Bed—One Assistant
  Procedure 22 Transferring the Patient from Chair to Bed—Two Assistants
  Procedure 23 Independent Transfer, Standby Assist
  Procedure 24 Transferring the Patient from Bed to Stretcher
  Procedure 25 Transferring the Patient from Stretcher to Bed
  Procedure 26 Transferring the Patient with a Mechanical Lift
  Procedure 27 Transferring the Patient onto and off the Toilet
  Procedure 28 Transferring the Patient into and out of the Bathtub
  Procedure 29 Transferring the Patient into and out of a Car

UNIT SUMMARY

Assisting patients to make transfers safely is an important nursing assistant function. There are basically two types of transfers:
- Sitting transfers.
- Standing transfers.

The type of transfer ordered depends on the patient's:
- Strength, endurance, and balance.
- Mental condition.
- Size.

Equipment used to facilitate transfers includes:
- Transfer belts.
- Mechanical lifts.

Transfers must be carried out smoothly, using proper body mechanics, to assure comfort and safety to both patient and worker.

NURSING ASSISTANT ALERT

Action	Benefit
Check equipment before using.	Unsafe equipment can be replaced and injury avoided.
Be sure bed and wheelchair or stretcher are locked before transfer.	Prevents potential accidents, injury, and deformity.
Explain procedure before transfer.	Enables patient to assist if possible.
Evaluate situation and get help if needed.	Reduces patient fears. Avoids injury to patient and staff.
Use proper transfer techniques.	Avoids injury to patient and caregiver.

ACTIVITIES

Vocabulary Exercise. Complete each sentence using the best term. Select terms from the list provided.

dependent   full weight   gait   paralyzed

partial weight   pivot   self   sitting

1. A mechanical lift may be used to transfer a _____ patient.

2. A patient who is able to stand on both legs is called _____ bearing.

3. The ability to stand on one leg is called _____ bearing.

4. A _____ patient does not have the ability to move.

5. A transfer belt is also called a _____ belt.

6. To _____ means to turn the entire body to one side.

Completion. Complete the statements in the spaces provided.

7. Before attempting to move or lift a patient, always determine if _____ is needed.

8. Before transferring a patient from bed to chair, you should know whether the patient is _____ bearing.

9. When assisting the patient from bed to wheelchair, make sure the chair is facing the _____ of the bed, and that the foot pedals are _____ .

10. When moving a patient with a mechanical lift, make sure the sling is positioned from _____ to _____ .

11. Four people should be positioned to move an unconscious person from a stretcher to bed as follows:

_____

_____

_____

_____

Corrections. Correct the statements that are wrong by crossing out the incorrect word or words. Write the correct words under them. Do not make any changes in the correct statements.

12. Know a patient's capabilities before attempting a transfer.

_____

13. Allow patients to place their hands around your neck.

_____

14. Use a lift sheet for standing transfers.

_____

15. Always explain the transfer plan to the patient.

_____

16. Transfer patients toward their weakest side.

_____

17. Patient shoes should have smooth soles and heels.

_____

18. Placing your hands under the patient's arms is acceptable during transfers.

_____

19. IVs, drainage bags, and other items must be considered during a transfer.

_____

20. Give the patient who is transferring only the assistance he needs.

_____

21. Before making a transfer, the bed should be in the high horizontal position.

_____

22. Always use correct body mechanics when making transfers.
23. During transfer, encourage the patient to focus his eyes on your hands.

_____

24. Stand close to the patient during a transfer.

_____

True/False. Mark the following true or false by circling T or F.

25. T F A transfer belt is used to assist patients to transfer.
26. T F A transfer belt can be used to lift a patient who has no ability to bear weight.
27. T F A transfer belt should be applied under the patient's clothing.
28. T F Always apply a transfer belt with the patient lying on his side.
29. T F The buckle of the transfer belt should be positioned in the front.
30. T F The transfer belt should be positioned around a female patient's breasts.
31. T F The transfer belt should be held using an underhand grasp.
32. T F The use of a transfer belt is contraindicated for a patient with abdominal aneurysm.
33. T F The transfer belt can be removed after the transfer is complete.
34. T F The transfer belt should be very tight.

Clinical Situations. Briefly describe how a nursing assistant should react in the following situations.

35. There is no one available in the radiology department when you arrive. You need help to move a patient. _____

_____

36. Your heavy patient is unable to help himself. He has returned from physical therapy and needs to be returned to bed. _____

_____

37. You must assist one other person to transfer a conscious patient from a stretcher to bed following an x-ray. _____

_____

_____

_____

38. You are assigned to transfer a patient to a chair using a mechanical lift. The sling is frayed where it hooks onto the lift frame.

_____

_____

39. Mr. Dunn is able to be up but is unstable when standing. He needs to empty his bladder._____

_____

Identification. Look carefully at each picture. List the corrections that should be made in each.

40.

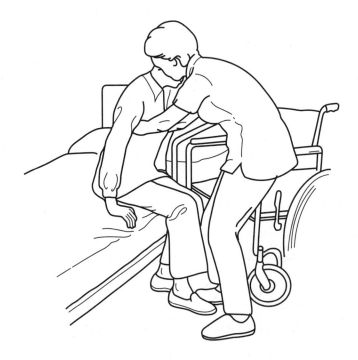

Corrections

    a. _____

    b. _____

    c. _____

41.

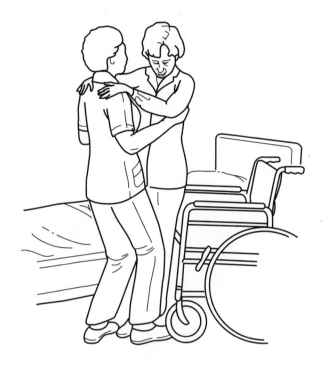

Corrections

    a. _____

    b. _____

    c. _____

42.

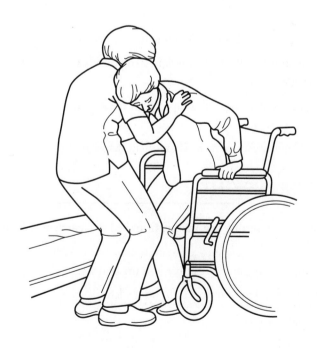

Corrections

    a. _____

    b. _____

    c. _____

43.

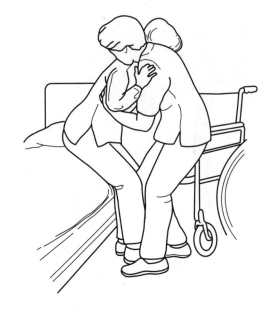

Corrections

a. _____

b. _____

c. _____

RELATING TO THE NURSING PROCESS

Write the step of the nursing process that is related to the nursing assistant action.

Nursing Assistant Action	**Nursing Process Step**
44. The nursing assistant carefully applies the transfer belt.	_____
45. The nursing assistant reports that the patient weighs 216 pounds and is paralyzed on the right side.	_____
46. The nursing assistant assembles all needed equipment at the bedside before attempting a transfer.	_____
47. The nursing assistant carefully checks the mechanical lift before using it.	_____

DEVELOPING GREATER INSIGHT

48. With classmates, practice transferring one another from bed to chair using one and then two assistants. Follow the special directions.

    a. Patient: put one arm in a sling and do not use it in the transfer.

    b. Patient: stand on right foot but bear no weight on the left.

49. Apply a transfer belt that is

    a. too loose.

    b. too tight.

50. Practice using a mechanical lift. Select a student to act as the patient.

51. Discuss why, when assisting a patient to get up or down, the patient should not place his or her hands on the body of the nursing assistant.

UNIT 16   The Patient's Mobility: Ambulation

OBJECTIVES

As a result of this unit, you will be able to:
- Spell and define terms.
- Describe the purpose of assistive devices used in ambulation.
- List safety measures for using assistive devices.
- Describe safety measures for using a wheelchair.
- Describe nursing assistant actions for:

  Ambulating a patient using a gait belt.
  Propelling a patient in a wheelchair.
  Positioning a patient in a wheelchair.
- Demonstrate the following procedures:

  Procedure 30 Assisting the Patient to Walk with a Cane and Three-Point Gait
  Procedure 31 Assisting the Patient to Walk with a Walker and Three-Point Gait
  Procedure 32 Assisting the Falling Patient

UNIT SUMMARY

Nursing assistants frequently assist patients with ambulation. Ambulating with assistance may require the use of an assistive device. Such assistive devices include:
- Gait belt.
- Walkers.
- Canes.

Nursing assistants must be competent in applying and using assistive devices safely.
Patients also will be transported in wheelchairs and correct techniques must be used.
Nursing assistants need to follow the appropriate procedure if a patient falls.

NURSING ASSISTANT ALERT

Action	Benefit
Apply assistive devices carefully and correctly.	Contributes to patients stability.
Use proper body mechanics when assisting a patient.	Avoids injury to patient and nursing assistant.

Action	Benefit
Learn the proper technique of two- and three-point gaits.	Provides knowledgeable support to patients using canes and walkers.
Know and practice proper care and use of wheelchairs.	Avoids accidents and injury to patients.

ACTIVITIES

Vocabulary Exercise. Write the words that form the circle on the left and their definitions on the right.

	Word	Definition
1.	_____	_____
2.	_____	_____
3.	_____	_____
4.	_____	_____
5.	_____	_____

Completion. Complete the following statements in the spaces provided. Select terms from the list provided.

affected	ambulation	arms	ball	four	heel
joint	need	rails	right	shoes	spills
strong	swinging	unsafe	90		

6. Walking is also known as _____ .

7. In normal walking, the _____ strikes the floor before the _____ of the foot.

8. During walking, the arms normally have a slight _____ movement.

9. To walk safely, the patient must have adequate _____ motion.

10. The type of assistive device selected depends upon a particular patient's _____ .

11. Patients should be encouraged to use hand _____ when walking.

12. When walking with a patient, the nursing assistant should stand on the patient's _____ side.

13. The nursing assistant should always check floors for clutter or _____ .

14. No assistive device should be used if it is _____ .

15. When forearm crutches with platforms are used, the elbows are in a constant _____-degree angle to the shoulder.

16. When patients ambulate, clothes should not hang down over the _____ .

17. A patient needs strength in both _____ to safely use a walker.

18. When ambulating with a walker, the patient shifts weight to the _____ leg as the walker is lifted and moved forward.

19. A properly fitting wheelchair will have about _____ inches between the top of the back and the patient's axillae.

20. When the feet are on the footrests of a wheelchair, the feet should be at _____ angles to the legs.

True/False. Mark the following true or false by circling T or F.

21. T   F   The arthritic patient has involuntary movements disturbing balance.

22. T   F   Protheses are used by patients who have had amputations to aid mobility.

23. T   F   Before initiating an ambulation program, a physical therapist evaluates the patient.

24. T   F   If a patient needs assistance but is using a cane, a gait belt need not be used.

25. T   F   Quad canes provide a narrow base of support.

26. T   F   Canes are recommended for aiding balance rather than providing support.

27. T   F   A walker should be narrow so the patient can walk behind it.

28. T   F   The walker can be used as a safe transfer device.

29. T   F   Patients who are ambulating with a walker may use a two-point or three-point gait.

30. T   F   A wheelchair that fits the patient properly will have a two- to three-inch clearance between the front edge of the seat and the back of the patient's knees.

Brief Answers. Briefly answer the statements in the spaces provided.

31. List six disorders that may affect a person's gait.

   a. _____   d. _____

   b. _____   e. _____

   c. _____   f. _____

32. Identify abilities that must be evaluated by a therapist before an ambulation program may be started.

   a. _____

   b. _____

   c. _____

   d. _____

   e. _____

   f. _____

   g. _____

33. Name three commonly used assistive devices.

   a. _____

   b. _____

   c. _____

34. Explain why standard crutches are seldom recommended for older adults. _____

_____

35. Explain the value of encouraging patients to carry out wheelchair push-ups.

_____

Clinical Situations. Briefly describe how a nursing assistant should react to the following situations.

36. Mrs. Keane is post-stroke and weak on her left side. She uses a walker when walking. You note that the hand grip is cracked and one of the bolt nuts is missing. _____

_____

37. Mr. Jacks is using a walker for stability because he is still weak following abdominal surgery for colon cancer. You notice he seems fatigued after walking the length of the corridor away from his room._____

_____

38. Mrs. De Koniger is ambulating with her walker. As she moves across the room, she moves her walker 15 inches in front of her, putting her weight on her weak leg as she brings her strong foot forward.

_____

_____

Identification.

39. Circle the letter of the figure below that shows the proper way to approach a closed door with a wheelchair.

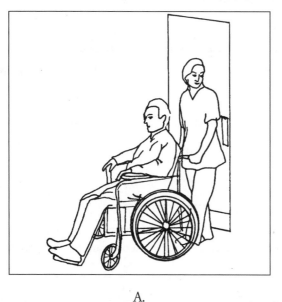
A.

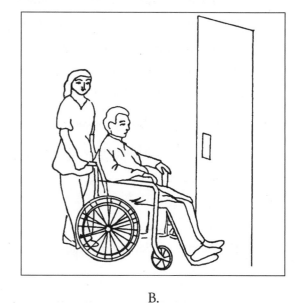
B.

RELATING TO THE NURSING PROCESS

Write the step of the nursing process that is related to the nursing assistant action.

Nursing Assistant Action	Nursing Process Step
40. Two nursing assistants use a small sheet under the patient's buttocks to move the patient up in his wheelchair.	_____
41. The nursing assistant reports to the nurse that the patient wishes to ambulate but only has poorly fitting slippers at the bedside.	_____
42. The nursing assistant uses alcohol and cotton swabs to clean debris out of the ridges of a cane tip.	_____
43. The nursing assistant picks up old newspapers from the floor and disposes of them.	_____

DEVELOPING GREATER INSIGHT

44. Try sitting in a wheelchair for one hour. Discuss your reaction and concerns with your classmates.

45. Gather different types of assistive devices. Practice using them yourself. Discuss any problems with your instructor.

46. Select one student to be the patient and others to be nursing assistants. Practice assisting the patient who has slipped down in the wheelchair to be properly aligned.

SECTION 6   MEASURING AND RECORDING VITAL SIGNS, HEIGHT, AND WEIGHT

UNIT 17   Body Temperature

OBJECTIVES

As a result of this unit, you will be able to:

■ Spell and define terms.

■ Name and identify the three types of clinical thermometers and tell their uses.

■ Read a thermometer.

■ Identify the range of normal values.

■ Demonstrate the following procedures:

Procedure 33 Measuring an Oral Temperature (Glass Thermometer)
Procedure 34 Measuring Temperature Using a Sheath-Covered Thermometer
Procedure 35 Measuring a Rectal Temperature (Glass Thermometer)
Procedure 36 Measuring an Axillary or Groin Temperature (Glass Thermometer)
Procedure 37 Measuring an Oral Temperature (Electronic Thermometer)
Procedure 38 Measuring a Rectal Temperature (Electronic Thermometer)
Procedure 39 Measuring an Axillary Temperature (Electronic Thermometer)
Procedure 40 Measuring a Tympanic Temperature
Procedure 41 Cleaning Glass Thermometers

UNIT SUMMARY

■ Temperature is the measurement of body heat. It varies in different areas in the same person.

Average oral temperature is 98.6°F.
Average rectal temperature is 99.6°F.
Average axillary temperature is 97.6°F.

■ Measurements of temperature may be made using the Fahrenheit (F) or Celsius (C) scale.

■ Three kinds of clinical thermometers are commonly used to measure the body temperature. They are the:

Oral.
Security.
Rectal.

■ There are different colored thermometer tips for rectal and oral use.

■ In addition to glass thermometers, there are other types of thermometers. They are the:

Battery-operated electronic thermometer. It has different colored tips for rectal and oral use.
Plastic thermometer. It has dots that change color according to the body temperature.
Tympanic thermometer. A probe placed in the external auditory canal measures body temperature at the tympanic membrane.
Digital thermometer. A probe is placed into the patient's mouth or rectum. It is battery-operated and the reading is shown as a digital display.

■ The procedure for measuring body temperature should be carefully followed, including beginning procedure and procedure completion activities.

NURSING ASSISTANT ALERT

Action	Benefit
Identify temperature values expressed in Fahrenheit scale.	Avoids error in measuring and recording temperature.
Be familiar with norms of temperature in different part of the body.	Proper nursing actions can be taken when abnormal values are identified.
Hold glass and rectal, digital, tympanic, and axillary thermometers and probes in place.	Ensures accurate temperature and avoids patient injury.
Be sure thermometers or probes are intact before insertion.	Prevents injury to the patient.
Record and report results accurately.	Ensures proper communication and evaluation of patient condition.

ACTIVITIES

Vocabulary Exercise. Define the words in the spaces provided.

1. body core _____

2. body shell _____

3. probe _____

4. tympanic _____

5. vital signs _____

Completion. Complete the statements in the spaces provided.

6. The measurement of body heat is called _____

7. Measurement of body heat is one of the vital signs. Name three others.

    a. _____

    b. _____

    c. _____

8. List eight factors that can influence body temperature.

    a. _____

    b. _____

    c. _____

    d. _____

    e. _____

    f. _____

    g. _____

    h. _____

9. In healthy adults, what is the usual daily variation in temperature?

10. When compared to adult body temperature, the temperature of children is _____ stable.

11. When using an electronic thermometer, which part is inserted into the patient?

_____

12. How is the part named in the previous question protected?

_____

13. What happens to the protector after use?_____

14. Glass thermometers are long cylindrical tubes that have a column of _____.

15. Each long line on a calibrated oral thermometer indicates an elevation of temperature of _____.

16. Each short line on the same thermometer indicates a rise in temperature of _____.

17. Three principles to keep in mind when reading a glass clinical thermometer are:

a. _____

b. _____

c. _____

18. If the mercury column ends between two lines, it should be read to the _____.

19. Write the names of the two scales used to measure a temperature.

a. _____

b. _____

20. What action should you take if the patient has just been smoking, drinking, or eating?

_____

21. Before inserting a clean thermometer into the patient's mouth, you should

a. _____

b. _____

c. _____

22. List three advantages of the tympanic thermometer.

a. _____

b. _____

c. _____

23. Indicate which method of temperature determination is best in each of the following circumstances (oral or rectal) if only glass thermometers are available.

Method

a. patient has diarrhea   _____

b. patient is confused   _____

c. patient cannot breathe through his nose   _____

d. patient has rectal bleeding   _____

e. patient is comatose   _____

f. patient has hemorrhoids   _____

g. patient is restless   _____

h. patient is a child   _____

i. patient has fecal impaction   _____

j. patient is coughing   _____

24. Name two areas other than the mouth or rectum that can be used to determine body temperature.

a. _____

b. _____

25. Thermometers must be left in place for the proper times to ensure recording. Write the time needed with each technique.

a. oral (glass thermometer) _____

b. rectal (glass thermometer) _____

c. groin (glass thermometer) _____

d. tympanic thermometer _____

e. digital rectal thermometer _____

26. Read the temperature measurement of each of the following glass thermometers.

Temperature Reading and Scale

a. _____

b. _____

c. _____

d. _____

e. _____

f. _____

g. _____

h. _____

i. _____

j. _____

a. 94 96 98 100 102 104 106 108 110

b. 94 96 98 100 102 104 106 108 110

c. 34 35 36 37 38 39 40 41 42 43

d. 94 96 98 100 102 104 106 108 110

e. 34 35 36 37 38 39 40 41 42 43

f. 94 96 98 100 102 104 106 108 110

g. 94 96 98 100 102 104 106 108 110

h. 34 35 36 37 38 39 40 41 42 43

i. 94 96 98 100 102 104 106 108 110

j. 34 35 36 37 38 39 40 41 42 43

27. Write the names of the thermometers pictured.

a. _____

b. _____

c. _____

d. _____

True/False. Mark the following true or false by circling T or F.

28. T F The body temperature is lower the closer to the body surface it is measured.

29. T F Body temperature is more stable in children than in adults.

30. T   F   The same person may have different temperatures when the temperature is determined from different parts of the body.

31. T   F   Hydration levels have no effect on body temperature.

32. T   F   Body heat is managed by special cells in the liver.

33. T   F   The bulb of a rectal thermometer should always be lubricated before insertion.

34. T   F   Used glass thermometers should always be washed in hot soapy water before disinfection.

35. T   F   A new disposable probe cover should be used on electronic thermometers with each patient.

36. T   F   The probe of the tympanic thermometer should be placed directly under the patient's tongue.

37. T   F   A patient's temperature should be recorded as soon as it is taken.

Clinical Situations.

38   Mrs. Morgan's oral temp was 98.4°F at 9 AM. When you see her at 10:30 AM she is flushed and her skin is dry. What action should you take?

39.   You are assigned to take the temperatures of two patients using the electronic thermometer and find the sheath package empty. You only have two temperatures to take and new sheaths are at the far end of the hall. What do you do?

RELATING TO THE NURSING PROCESS

Write the step of the nursing process that is related to the nursing assistant action.

Nursing Assistant Action	Nursing Process Step
40. The nursing assistant checks the glass thermometer carefully before placing it under the patient's tongue.	_____
41. The nursing assistant accurately reports that the patient's temperature is 102°F orally.	_____
42. Before inserting a mercury clinical thermometer, the nursing assistant makes sure the mercury reads below 96°F.	_____
43. The nursing assistant checks the nursing care plan before measuring an oral temperature when she notices the patient is receiving oxygen by face mask.	_____
44. The nursing assistant reports that the patient feels faint and has hot, flushed skin.	_____

DEVELOPING GREATER INSIGHT

45. Practice taking temperatures using different types of thermometers.

46. Discuss with your teacher and classmates why proper placement of the tympanic thermometer is important.

47. Think about the reasons disposable gloves are used for temperature-taking procedures.

48. Explain to classmates why glass clinical thermometers are wiped from tip toward bulb when removed from the patient.

UNIT 18   Pulse and Respiration

OBJECTIVES

As a result of this unit, you will be able to:
- Spell and define terms.
- Define pulse.
- Explain the importance of monitoring a pulse rate.
- Locate the pulse sites.
- Identify the range of normal pulse and respiratory rates.
- Measure the pulse at different locations.
- List the characteristics of pulse and respiration.
- Demonstrate the following procedures:
  Procedure 42 Counting the Radial Pulse
  Procedure 43 Counting the Apical-Radial Pulse
  Procedure 44 Counting Respirations

UNIT SUMMARY

- Pulse and respiration rates and character are determined as part of the vital signs.
- The values are usually determined in a single procedure.
- Differences in apical and radial pulse rates are known as pulse deficits.
- Accurate values for respirations are best obtained when the patient is unaware that the procedure is being carried out.
- Unusual findings should be reported to the nurse.

NURSING ASSISTANT ALERT

Action	Benefit
Measure and record the character of pulse and respiration.	Provides important information regarding patient condition.
Recognize factors that alter pulse or respiratory rate.	Factors may be taken into account when evaluating findings.
Identify the norms for pulse and respiratory rates.	Proper nursing assistant actions may be taken when abnormal findings are identified.
Record findings accurately.	Ensures proper communication and evaluation of patient condition to other health care providers.

ACTIVITIES

Vocabulary Exercise. Each line has four different spellings of a word. Circle the correctly spelled word.

1. appical   apical   apecal   apicale
2. cyanosis   sianosis   syanosis   cyanoses
3. poulse   pullse   polse   pulse
4. despnea   dypnea   disnea   dyspnia
5. apnea   epnea   apnia   appnea
6. tachipnea   tachypnea   takipnea   tachipnia
7. rhythm   rhythem   rhethem   rytham
8. bradekardia   bradicardea   bradycardia   bradykardya

Completion. Complete the following statements in the spaces provided.

9. The pulse is the _____ of blood felt against the wall of an _____ .

10. The pulse can be felt best in _____ that come close to the _____ and can be gently pressed against a _____ .

11. When the patient is unconscious, you should measure the _____ pulse.

12. Pulse measurement includes determining the pulse character, which means the _____ and _____ .

13. To check circulation to the toes of your patient with diabetes, you should palpate the _____ artery.

14. Seven major arteries used to measure pulse rates are:

    a. _____

    b. _____

    c. _____

    d. _____

    e. _____

    f. _____

    g. _____

15. In an adult the normal pulse rate is between _____ bpm and _____ bpm.

16. Ten factors that can alter the pulse rate are:

    a. _____

    b. _____

    c. _____

    d. _____

    e. _____

    f. _____

    g. _____

    h. _____

    i. _____

    j. _____

17. Your patient is 8 years old and has a pulse rate of 100. You know this is _____ for a child this age.

18. To accurately measure a pulse rate, your watch must have a _____ .

19. You should locate the pulse with your _____ .

20. The pulse should be counted for _____ .

True/False. Mark the following true or false by circling T or F.

21. T   F   Normally the apical pulse is 4 bpm greater than the radial in the same person.

22. T   F   Three health care providers are needed to accurately measure an apical pulse.

23. T   F   When determining an apical pulse, you will need a stethoscope.

24. T   F   The earpieces of the stethoscope must be cleaned before use.

25. T   F   Moist respirations are best documented as stertorous.

26. T   F   Each respiration consists of one inspiration and one expiration.

27. T   F   Symmetry of respirations refers to the depth of respiration.

28. T   F   The regularity of respirations is referred to as the rhythm.

29. T   F   The normal adult rate is 25 respirations per minute.

30. T   F   Always count the respiratory rate after you inform the patient of your action.

Clinical Situations. Briefly describe how a nursing assistant should react to the following situations.

31. You are measuring vital signs and notice the patient in 112B, whose pulse rate has been 84 to 88 bpm, now has a pulse rate of 112 and the pulse is weak.

   _____

32. Mr. Murray has a medical diagnosis of congestive heart failure. When you measure his pulse you find it irregular and weak. The nurse says she suspects a pulse deficit.

   _____

33. You report that Mr. Rossi has a pulse deficit of 24 and a pulse rate of 84. What was the patient's apical pulse, and how would you document the reading? Show your work.

   _____

34. Find the pulse deficit in each of the following readings and show proper documentation.

   a. apical pulse 120 radial pulse 104 _____

   b. apical pulse 118 radial pulse 88 _____

   c. apical pulse 92 radial pulse 50 _____

   d. apical pulse 102 radial pulse 68 _____

   e. apical pulse 98 radial pulse 76 _____

RELATING TO THE NURSING PROCESS

Write the step of the nursing process that is related to the nursing assistant action.

Nursing Assistant Action   **Nursing Process Step**

35. The nursing assistant tells the nurse that the patient's respirations have become more labored.

   _____

36. The nursing assistant has an order to determine the apical pulse. She seeks help because she is not sure how to perform this procedure.   _____

37. The patient's pulse rate is 60 and the nursing assistant reports this information to the nurse.   _____

38. The nursing assistant has difficulty hearing the blood pressure clearly and asks the nurse to help her.   _____

39. The nursing assistant listens closely as the nurse explains the new revised care plans for her patients.   _____

40. The nursing assistant listens and counts the respirations for a full minute when the patient's respirations are irregular   _____

DEVELOPING GREATER INSIGHT

41. Practice taking pulse and respiration readings on your classmates. Have your instructor check your findings.

42. Discuss with the class ways to handle the following situations:

    a. Mr. Volaire has an irregular pulse rate.

    b. Mrs. Benton has an IV in one wrist.

    c. Mrs. Zeldane seems to stop breathing each time you complete her pulse rate and begin to count her respirations.

    d. Mr. Capione has pulse and respiratory rates that have increased since your last measurement.

UNIT 19   Blood Pressure

OBJECTIVES

As a result of this unit, you will be able to:
- Spell and define terms.
- Describe the factors that influence blood pressure.
- Identify the range of normal blood pressure values.
- Identify the causes of inaccurate blood pressure readings.
- Select the proper size blood pressure cuff.
- List precautions associated with use of the sphygmomanometer.
- Demonstrate the following procedure:

  Procedure 45 Taking Blood Pressure

UNIT SUMMARY

Blood pressure must be determined and recorded accurately by watching the gauge of the sphygmomanometer and listening with the stethoscope.
- Note and record the first regular sound as the systolic pressure.
- Note and record the change sound or last sound as the diastolic pressure, as determined by facility policy.
- Recheck unusual readings after one minute.
- Report unusual blood pressure to the nurse.
- Document the blood pressure as an improper fraction with the systolic reading above the diastolic reading.

NURSING ASSISTANT ALERT

Action	Benefit
Use blood pressure cuff of proper size.	Correct readings can be obtained only if proper size cuff is used.
Clean stethoscope earpieces before and after use.	Prevents transmission of infection between caregivers.
Do not take blood pressure on an arm that is being infused or is paralyzed.	Prevents injury to the patient.
Read gauge at eye level.	Gives accurate reading.

ACTIVITIES

Vocabulary Exercise. Complete the puzzle by filling in the missing letters of words found in this unit. Use the definitions to help you discover these words.

1.   H   1.

2.   — Y — — — — — — — — —   2. high blood pressure

3.   — — P — — — — — — — —   3. drugs that slow down body
                                                                              function

4.   — — — — — E —   4. felt

5.   — R — — — — —   5. artery most often used to
                                                                              determine blood pressure

6.   — — — — T — — — — —   6. stretchability

7.   E   7.

8. — — — — — — — N — — — — —   8. blood pressure cuff and gauge

9.   — — S — — — —   9. not eating

10.   — — — — — — I —   10. lowest blood pressure reading

11.   — — — — — — — O — —   11. an instrument used to hear
                                                                              body sounds

12.   — — — — — — N — —   12. drugs that speed up body
                                                                              functions

Completion. Complete the statements in the spaces provided.

13. Blood pressure depends on four factors. They are:

   a. _____

   b. _____

   c. _____

   d. _____

14. List five factors other than heredity that can cause an elevated blood pressure.

   a. _____

   b. _____

   c. _____

   d. _____

   e. _____

15. List five factors that can lower blood pressure, other than grief.

   a. _____

   b. _____

   c. _____

   d. _____

   e. _____

16. When selecting a blood pressure cuff, it should measure approximately _____ of the patient's arm.

17. Three types of sphygmomanometers in common use are:

a. _____

b. _____

c. _____

18. The patient has a blood pressure reading of 148/98. You recognize this as _____.

19. The difference between the systolic and diastolic pressure is called the _____.

20. Three reasons for not using an arm to measure blood pressure are: the arm is _____, the arm is the site of an _____ , or the arm is _____ .

21. Sound that fades out for 10 to 15 mm Hg and then resumes as you deflate the cuff is known as _____.

22. The large lines on the blood pressure gauge are at increments of _____ Hg.

23. Each small line on the blood pressure gauge indicates _____ intervals.

24. The cuff should be applied _____ above the elbow.

25. The center of the rubber bladder should be placed directly over the _____ .

26. Three situations that you should immediately report regarding blood pressure measurement are:

a. _____

b. _____

c. _____

27. Unusual blood pressure readings ought to be checked after _____.

28. Identify the equipment and the specific parts.

a. _____

b. _____

c. _____

d. _____

e. _____

f. _____

g. _____

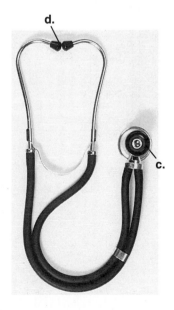

a.

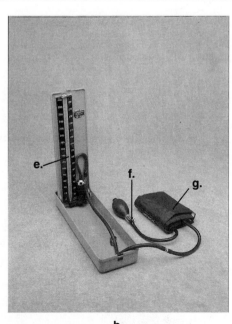

b.

29. Determine the systolic and diastolic readings.

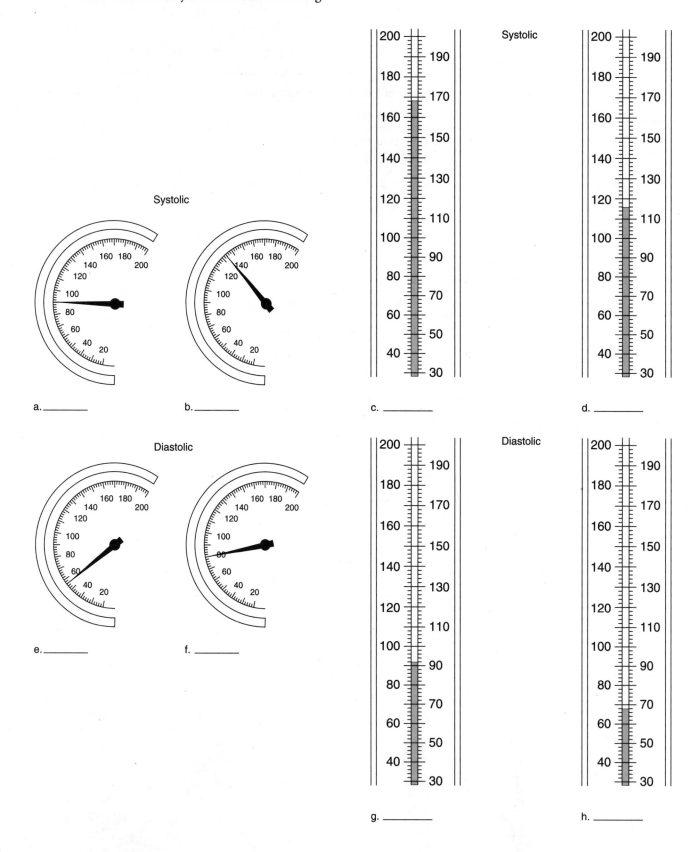

Systolic

a. _____   b. _____   c. _____   d. _____

Diastolic

e. _____   f. _____   g. _____   h. _____

True/False. Mark the following true or false by circling T or F.

30. T F   The same size blood pressure cuff may be used with all patients.

31. T F   The highest point of blood pressure measurement is the diastolic reading.

32. T F   Hereditary factors can cause an elevated blood pressure.

33. T F   Deflating the cuff too slowly can result in an inaccurate reading.

34. T F   All blood pressure readings should be made with the gauge above eye level.

35. T F   The diastolic pressure is measured at the change sound or last sound that is heard.

36. T F   The blood pressure is most often taken over the brachial artery.

37. T F   Always clean the stethoscope earpieces and diaphragm before and after use.

38. T F   Grief lowers the blood pressure.

39. T F   Blood pressure readings are always recorded as a proper fraction such as 40/110.

40. T F   It is very important to use a cuff of the proper size when determining the blood pressure.

41. T F   A blood pressure may be measured using an arm that is being infused.

RELATING TO THE NURSING PROCESS

Write the step of the nursing process that is related to the nursing assistant action.

Nursing Assistant Action	Nursing Process Step
42. The nursing assistant finds that the patient's blood pressure is higher than the previous reading and reports this information.	_____
43. The patient is very heavy and the nursing assistant seeks guidance as to which size blood pressure cuff to use.	_____
44. The nursing assistant informs the team leader of the patient's vital signs before leaving for a break.	_____

DEVELOPING GREATER INSIGHT

45. What action is taking place in the heart when you see the systolic reading?

46. Practice taking blood pressure on patients whose arms are different sizes.

47. A patient has polycythemia vera, a condition that increases the number of red blood cells. Explain what effect this condition has on the blood pressure.

48. Explain why narrowing of the blood vessels raises blood pressure.

49. Explain why a blood pressure cuff should not be placed on an arm with an IV inserted.

UNIT 20   Measuring Height and Weight

OBJECTIVES

As a result of this unit, you will be able to:
- Spell and define terms.
- Describe the proper use of an overbed scale.
- Demonstrate the following procedures:

Procedure 46   Weighing and Measuring the Patient Using an Upright Scale
Procedure 47   Weighing the Patient on a Chair Scale
Procedure 48   Measuring Weight with an Electronic Wheelchair Scale
Procedure 49   Measuring and Weighing the Patient in Bed

UNIT SUMMARY

Measurement of the patient's height and weight is usually taken on admission.
- Medications are often given according to the patient's weight.
- Weight changes may reflect the patient's condition and progress.

Measurements of height are made in:
- Feet (′).
- Inches (″).
- Centimeters (cm).

Measurements of weight are made in:
- Pounds (lb).
- Kilograms (kg).

Different techniques and equipment are used to make height and weight determinations depending on the patient's condition.

NURSING ASSISTANT ALERT

Action	Benefit
Recognize that weight may be recorded in pounds and kilograms.	Avoid errors in measuring and documenting weights.
Remember that height can be measured in feet, inches, and centimeters.	Ensures correct interpretation of findings.
Always balance the scale before using.	Ensures correct weight.

ACTIVITIES

Vocabulary Exercise. Put a circle around the word defined.

```
A C A L I B R A T E D F C K
H D I N C K E A V J M B S I
S L G S A D O G N H F R V L
M C E N T I M E T E R E N O
J O A T H F B P I L D P B G
P B A L A N C E B A R K Q R
E M B I E L A H E I G H T A
U I N C R E M E N T S L H M
G N A D Q F M B I K D O C J
P O U N D S E F I N C H E A
```

1. equal to 2.5 cm
2. length of a person
3. marked
4. amounts
5. equal to 2.2 pounds
6. increments measured by small indicator on scale
7. part of scale showing increments
8. device used to weigh a person

Completion. Complete the statements in the spaces provided. Select terms from the list provided.

bed	chair	clothing	empty	kilogram
metric	paper towel	same	scale	
sling	tape measure	upright	wheelchair	

9. Choose the correct scale for each patient.

   a. Mr. Graham is in a wheelchair and cannot stand. He should be weighed with a/an _____ scale.

   b. Mrs. Almos is recovering from pneumonia and is up and about as desired. She should be weighed with a/an _____ scale.

   c. Mrs. DerHagopian is elderly. Her condition requires constant bed rest. She should be weighed with a/an _____ scale.

10. Patients should be weighed at the _____ time each day.

11. Patients should wear the same type of _____ each time they are weighed.

12. The same method and _____ should be used each time a patient is weighed.

13. Patients should _____ their bladders before weighing.

14. When a patient cannot get out of bed, height measurement may be made with a _____ .

15. Before weighing a patient, the platform of an upright scale should be covered with a _____ .

16. Some facilities use the _____ system, which records weights in _____ .

Reading Weights and Heights. Read each weight measurement and record it in pounds.

17. _____

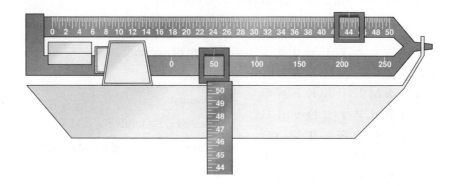

18. _____

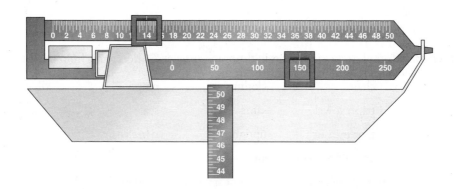

19. _____

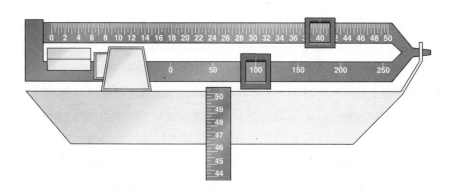

20. _____

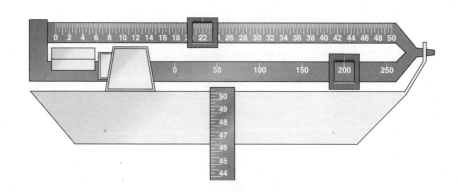

Read each height measurement and record it in feet and inches.

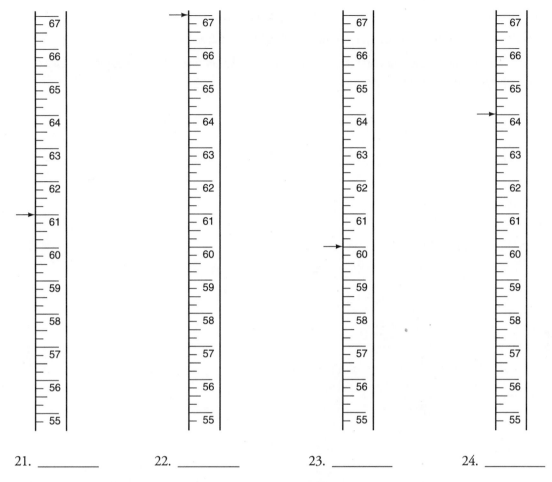

21. _____   22. _____   23. _____   24. _____

True/False. Mark the following true or false by circling T or F.

25. T   F   Weights should be moved to the extreme left before weighing.

26. T   F   Patients may hold the bar while being weighed as long as they do not lean on the scale.

27. T   F   Before weighing a patient on a wheelchair scale, be sure to weigh the wheelchair only.

28. T   F   The wheels of a wheelchair need not be locked when weighing the patient on a wheelchair scale.

29. T   F   When using a sling scale, the patient's body must be completely free of the bed before a reading is taken.

RELATING TO THE NURSING PROCESS

Write the step of the nursing process that is related to the nursing assistant action.

Nursing Assistant Action	Nursing Process Step
30. The nursing assistant measures and weighs the new patient as instructed.	_____
31. The nursing assistant reports information about the patient's height and weight to the team leader and records it on the patient's record.	_____

DEVELOPING GREATER INSIGHT

32. With classmates, practice the safe use of different types of scales.

33. Explain why a patient whose height is 64 inches is recorded as 5 feet 4 inches.

34. Mrs. Menitt is a new admission. She cannot get out of bed. Think through the steps you will take to obtain a correct height measurement.

UNIT 21   Admission, Transfer, and Discharge

OBJECTIVES

As a result of this unit, you will be able to:
- Spell and define terms.
- List the ways the nursing assistant can help in the processes of admission, transfer and discharge.
- Demonstrate the following procedures:

  Procedure 50 Admitting the Patient
  Procedure 51 Transferring the Patient
  Procedure 52 Discharging the Patient

UNIT SUMMARY

The nursing assistant has specific responsibilities related to the admission, transfer, and discharge of the patient. These responsibilities include:
- Providing emotional support to both patient and family.
- Assisting in the safe physical transport of the patient.
- Carrying out the specific procedures relating to admission, transfer, and discharge.
- Preparing and disassembling the patient unit before and after use.
- Reporting and documenting observations.

NURSING ASSISTANT ALERT

Action	Benefit
Consider needs of visitors as well as those of the new patient.	Contributes to patient and family feelings of welcome and security.
Make careful observations and accurate documentation.	Provides information essential to the formulation of an appropriate nursing care plan.

ACTIVITIES

Vocabulary Exercise. Write the words forming the circle and define them. Start at the arrow.

TRANSFERDISCHARGEBASELINEASSESSMENTADMISSION

1. _____

2. _____

3. _____

4. _____

5. _____

Completion. Complete the statements in the spaces provided.

6. Admission to a care facility is a cause of great concern for both _____ and _____ .

7. The nursing assistant should identify the patient by speaking her name and

_____ .

8. Jewelry and valuables not left at the cashier's office should be _____ , signed for, and sent home.

9. The nursing assistant can help orient the patient to the unit by explaining how to use the phone or television and the times _____ are served.

10. When transferring a patient to another unit, your manner should be _____ and efficient.

11. Never leave the patient, his records, or medications _____ during the transfer procedure.

12. After a transfer is completed, you should be sure the patient is _____ and _____ .

13. Before preparing the patient for discharge, make sure the _____ has been written.

14. The nursing assistant's _____ are very valuable in the nurse's baseline assessment.

15. The patient is the facility's _____ until she has left the building.

16. After discharge, a final _____ is made on the patient chart.

17. Before the patient leaves for discharge, make sure the _____ have been given to him.

18. DRGs were introduced for the purpose of _____ .

Brief Answers. Briefly answer the statements in the spaces provided.

19. The admission kit includes:

a. _____

b. _____

c. _____

d. _____

e. _____

f. _____

20. The nursing assistant can facilitate the admission procedure if seven points are kept in mind and carried out. List them.

a. _____

b. _____

c. _____

d. _____

e. _____

f. _____

g. _____

21. Before admitting the patient you will need specific information. What questions should you ask the nurse?

a. _____

b. _____

c. _____

Clinical Situations. Briefly describe how a nursing assistant should react to the following situations.

22. Your patient tells you he intends to leave the health care facility without his physician's permission.

_____

23. Your patient has just been discharged.

_____

_____

_____

24. The family accompanies your patient to the unit and must wait as you carry out the admission procedure. How can you show courtesy to them?

_____

_____

_____

_____

_____

25. Your assignment is to admit the patient to Room 16C. Explain the equipment you will gather.

_____

_____

_____

_____

_____

RELATING TO THE NURSING PROCESS

Write the step of the nursing process that is related to the nursing assistant action.

Nursing Assistant Action	Nursing Process Step
26. The nursing assistant carefully prepares the patient's unit before admission.	_____
27. The nursing assistant measures the vital signs during the admission procedure.	_____
28. During admission the nursing assistant carefully observes the patient and listens to the patient's statements.	_____
29. The nursing assistant makes sure that all the patient's personal articles are transported to the new unit when the patient is transferred.	_____
30. The nursing assistant documents the correct time and method of patient discharge on the proper record.	_____

DEVELOPING GREATER INSIGHT

31. With classmates, role-play the following situations (consider equipment, psychological, and physical needs):

    a. Mrs. Coe is being admitted. She is in a wheelchair and very frail.

    b. Mr. Fletcher is ambulatory and is being discharged to the care of his son and daughter-in-law. The daughter-in-law seems very nervous and is pacing back and forth.

    c. Mrs. Barkley spends most of the day in a wheelchair. She is to be transferred to another floor.

UNIT 22   Bedmaking

OBJECTIVES

As a result of this unit, you will be able to:
- Spell and define terms.
- List the different types of beds and their uses.
- Operate each type of bed.
- Properly handle clean and soiled linens.
- Demonstrate the following procedures:

  Procedure 53 Making a Closed Bed
  Procedure 54 Opening the Closed Bed
  Procedure 55 Making an Occupied Bed
  Procedure 56 Making the Surgical Bed

UNIT SUMMARY

Proper bedmaking is an important part of your work.
- A skillfully made bed provides comfort and safety for the patient.
- Beds may be built to meet specific patient needs and conditions. Each type of bed will be made differently.
- Types of beds include:

  CircOlectric® bed.
  Stryker frame.
  Clinitron®.
  Electric.
  Gatch.
- Bedmaking methods include:

  Closed bed.
  Occupied bed.
  Unoccupied bed.
  Surgical bed.
- Drawsheets or turning sheets may be used, depending on patient requirements.
- Some facilities use fitted bottom sheets. The bedmaking procedure may be changed to accommodate this difference.

NURSING ASSISTANT ALERT

Action	Benefit
Handle linen carefully and properly.	Prevents spread of germs.
Raise bed to comfortable working height during procedure.	Reduces strain on caregiver.
Make bed neatly and smoothly.	Contributes to comfort and lessens chance of (pressure) ulcer formation.
Know how to operate bed and equipment before attempting to do so.	Avoids injury to patient and caregiver.
Always leave bed in lowest horizontal position.	Lessens the possibility of accidents when patient gets in and out of bed.
Use standard precautions if contact with blood, body fluids, secretions, or excretions is likely.	Prevents spread of germs. Protects caregiver.

ACTIVITIES

Vocabulary Exercise. Unscramble the words introduced in this unit and define them.

1. YRTRESK   _____

2. HACGT   _____

3. TSOBXEPAL   _____

4. IETDREM   _____

5. FFAONLD   _____

6. IRSEADLIS   _____

7. ETHES   _____

True/False. Mark the following true or false by circling T or F.

8. T F A patient suffering from a spinal cord injury would most likely be placed on a Stryker frame or CircOlectric® bed.

9. T F After the bottom of the bed has been made, you then pull the mattress to the head of the bed.

10. T F Before making a bed, lower it to its lowest horizontal height.

11. T F When completing an open bed, the top bedding is positioned to the top of the bed under the pillow.

12. T F The top linen of a surgical bed is left untucked and fanfolded to one side.

13. T F A lift sheet should be positioned from the patient's waist to his knees.

14. T F The electrically operated bed is the most common type of bed found in an acute care facility.

15. T F In most facilities a licensed nurse must be present when a nursing assistant turns a patient on a circle bed.

16. T F A mattress pad is applied to the mattress before the bottom sheet.

17. T F Fitted sheets are used in some facilities in place of top sheets.

18. T F Before making an unoccupied bed, arrange the linen in the order it is to be used.

19. T F Always position a patient comfortably before leaving the room.

20. T F The flat bottom sheet should be placed so the bottom edge is even with the end of the mattress at the foot of the bed.

21. T F Linen to make a bed should be placed on the overbed table.

22. T F Never shake the linen when making a bed, because this may spread germs.

23. T F When making the bottom of an occupied bed, the linen should be rolled against the patient's back and then tucked under the patient's body.

24. T F The top linen should be loosened when bed is occupied.

25. T F Side rails should be up and secure before you leave an occupied bed.

Identification. Name the type of corner that has been made in the top linen.

26. a. _____

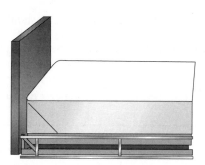

b. _____

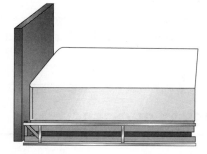

Brief Answers. Briefly answer the following questions.

27. Why should one side of the bed be made at a time?

_____

28. Why are the sheets unfolded rather than shaken out?

_____

29. How should the pillow be placed on the bed?

_____

30. What is the purpose of the open bed?

_____

31. What is the purpose of the surgical bed?

_____

32. Why is it important to screen the patient unit before beginning to make an occupied bed?

_____

33. What must be the position of the bed and side rails of the occupied bed before leaving?

_____

34. What is the proper position for the overbed table when the bed is closed or unoccupied?

_____

35. When is the closed bed made in the hospital?

_____

36. Why would the wheels of the bed be locked before the nursing assistant starts to make the bed?

_____

Clinical Situations. Briefly describe how a nursing assistant should react to the following situations.

37. You finish making the occupied bed and you notice the bed is at the working horizontal height. _____

_____

38. Your patient is in a CircOlectric® bed and you have never operated this kind of bed.

_____

_____

39. A visitor tells you that her father is to be placed on a Clinitron® bed and asks you what kind of bed that is.

_____

_____

_____

40. You took an extra clean towel that was not needed after you entered the patient's room. What should be done with the towel?

_____

RELATING TO THE NURSING PROCESS

Write the step of the nursing process that is related to the nursing assistant action.

Nursing Assistant Action	Nursing Process Step
41. The nursing assistant makes sure the bottom bed linen is free of wrinkles.	_____
42. The nursing assistant accompanies the nurse so the assistant can assist in turning a patient on a CircOlectric® bed.	_____
43. The nursing assistant makes sure the patient is not exposed when he changes the bed linen.	_____

44. The nursing assistant is assigned to prepare a bed for a postoperative patient. Because she has not done this before, she asks the nurse for clarification. _____

DEVELOPING GREATER INSIGHT

45. Wrinkle the bottom linen on a bed. Make sure there are wrinkles. Put on your nightwear and spend 20 minutes on the wrinkles.

46. Make the top linen very tight. Be sure to tuck in the top sheet and spread tightly. Spend 20 minutes in this bed.

47. Discuss with classmates the reasons why making beds would be very fatiguing if proper procedures were not followed.

48. Discuss with classmates the importance of using a foam wedge at the head of the bed with an alternating-pressure mattress when the patient eats.

UNIT 23 Patient Bathing

OBJECTIVES

As a result of this unit, you will be able to:
- Spell and define terms.
- Describe the safety precautions for patient bathing.
- List the purposes of bathing patients.
- State the value of whirlpool baths.
- Demonstrate the following procedures:

    Procedure 57 Assisting with the Tub Bath or Shower
    Procedure 58 Bed Bath
    Procedure 59 Partial Bath
    Procedure 60 Female Perineal Care
    Procedure 61 Male Perineal Care
    Procedure 62 Hand and Fingernail Care
    Procedure 63 Bed Shampoo
    Procedure 64 Dressing and Undressing Patient

UNIT SUMMARY

Bathing makes a patient feel refreshed and clean. Full or partial baths may be carried out in:
- Bed.
- Showers.
- Regular bathtub.
- Whirlpool tub.

Personal hygiene measures include care of the:
- Teeth.
- Hair.
- Nails.
- Dressing and Undressing.

Patients should be encouraged to participate in personal hygiene measures and the choice of garments.
Range-of-motion exercises are frequently performed during the bath procedure, according to the patient's needs and orders. See Unit 38. The daily hygiene routine gives you a chance to make close observations of the patient.

NURSING ASSISTANT ALERT

Action	Benefit
Guard against falls.	Avoids potential injury.
Maintain an even room temperature.	Prevents chilling and discomfort.
Avoid unnecessary exposure.	Protects patient's dignity and privacy.
Work quickly and smoothly, using proper body mechanics.	Lessens patient and caregiver fatigue

ACTIVITIES

Vocabulary Exercise. Each line has four different spellings of a word. Circle the correctly spelled word.

1. cutical   cuticule   cuticale   cuticle
2. axillae   axiller   axella   arxilla
3. genetala   genitalia   genetalea   ginetalia
4. middriff   medrif   midriff   midreff
5. pubic   pubec   pobic   paobic

Completion. Complete the statements in the spaces provided.

6. A daily bath makes the patient feel _____ , and clean.

7. In addition to bathing the body, morning care includes cleaning the teeth, _____ , and _____ .

8. A partial bath ensures cleansing of the hands, face, _____ , buttocks, and _____ .

9. The best temperature for bath water is about _____ °F.

10. A _____ should be in the bath area in case of an emergency.

11. After the tub bath is completed and the patient has returned to the unit, return to the tub room and _____ the tub.

12. To provide privacy during a tub bath or shower, the patient may use a _____ to wrap around his _____ .

13. As the patient steps out of the tub, hold a _____ around the patient to provide privacy.

14. During a bed bath, privacy can be provided by _____ .

15. Before the bed bath, you should offer the patient a _____ .

16. When preparing the patient for a bed bath, remove the top bedding and replace it with a

_____

17. Do not use soap near the _____ .

18. When cleaning the eyes, always wipe from _____ to _____ corner.

19. Pay special attention to the folds under a female patient's _____ as you wash her.

20. Powder should not be used because it is apt to _____ .

21. Apply _____ to the feet of a patient with dry skin.

22. When grooming the toenails, file _____ across and do not push back the _____ .

23. When finishing the bath for the male patient, carefully wash and dry the _____ ,
_____ , and groin area.

24. The whirlpool tub provides the beneficial action of a _____ in addition to cleaning.

25. When giving foot care, allow the feet to soak for _____ minutes.

26. Two abnormalities you might note during foot care are _____ and callouses.

27. When giving a bed shampoo, _____ the scalp with your _____ .

28. During a bed shampoo, give the patient a _____ to protect the patient's eyes.

29. Dry the hair following a shampoo with a _____ or portable hair dryer.

Brief Answers. Briefly answer the following questions.

30. Three values patients derive from a bath include:

a. _____

b. _____

c. _____

31. Three precautions you should take when the patient is able to bathe himself in a tub include:

a. _____

b. _____

c. _____

32. Special care must be given during the bath to the patient who:

a. _____

b. _____

c. _____

33. There are eleven procedure completion actions. They are:

a. _____

b. _____

c. _____

d. _____

e. _____

f. _____

g. _____

h. _____

i. _____

j. _____

k. _____

34. Describe how you should remove the gown of a patient receiving an intravenous infusion in order to bathe the patient.

   a. _____

   b. _____

   c. _____

   d. _____

   e. _____

   f. _____

35. Describe how a bath mitt is made.

   _____

   _____

   _____

36. Why should the patient help you with the bed bath as much as his condition permits?

   _____

37. What is the assistant's responsibility when the patient is unable to complete his bath?

   _____

38. What other procedures may be carried out in conjunction with the bath procedure?

   _____

39. What are four values of the whirlpool bath?

   a. _____

   b. _____

   c. _____

   d. _____

40. What measures can be taken to help avoid patient falls during tub bathing?

   _____

   _____

   _____

Clinical Situations. Briefly describe how a nursing assistant should react to the following situations.

41. Your patient feels weak or faint during a tub bath.

   _____

   _____

42. You have not yet finished bathing the legs of a bed patient and the water feels cool.

   _____

43. Your patient is a diabetic and his toenails need cutting.

   _____

44. Describe the technique to be used when washing the penis and scrotum.

   _____

RELATING TO THE NURSING PROCESS

Write the step of the nursing process that is related to the nursing assistant action.

Nursing Assistant Action   **Nursing Process Step**

45. The nursing assistant carefully cleans the tub before and after each patient use.   _____

46. The nursing assistant has to bathe a patient with an IV line and isn't sure
    how to remove the patient's gown. She asks a nurse for help.   _____

47. The nursing assistant offers a bedpan to the patient before giving a bed bath.   _____

48. The nursing assistant finds the patient cannot separate her legs sufficiently
    to provide good perineal care and asks the nurse for directions so that care
    can be given.   _____

49. The nursing assistant is giving foot care to a patient with thick long toenails.
    He asks the nurse if the nails should be cut.   _____

50. The nursing assistant listens carefully as the nurse explains that the care plan
    for a bed bath will be modified the next day to allow the patient to shower if she
    feels well enough.   _____

DEVELOPING GREATER INSIGHT

51. Discuss why frequent perineal care is important to the patient's hygiene.

52. Discuss why nursing assistants are not permitted to cut the toenails of a diabetic patient.

53. Discuss ways to give perineal care if the patient cannot separate his or her legs.

54. Working with another student, demonstrate the proper way to assist a person put on an undershirt that slips over
    the head when the patient cannot use one side of her body.

55. Think through the reason why you should be ready to assist patients put on shoes and socks.

UNIT 24   General Comfort Measures

OBJECTIVES

As a result of this unit, you will be able to:
- Spell and define terms.
- Discuss the reasons for early morning and bedtime care.
- Identify patients who require frequent oral hygiene.
- List the purposes of oral hygiene.
- Explain nursing assistant responsibilities for a patient's dentures.
- State the purpose of backrubs.
- Describe safety precautions when shaving a patient.
- Describe the important of his care.
- Explain the use of comfort devices.
- Demonstrate the following procedures:

  Procedure 65 Assisting with Routine Oral Hygiene
  Procedure 66 Assisting with Special Oral Hygiene
  Procedure 67 Assisting Patient to Floss and Brush Teeth
  Procedure 68 Caring for Dentures
  Procedure 69 Backrub
  Procedure 70 Shaving a Male Patient
  Procedure 71 Daily Hair Care
  Procedure 72 Giving and Receiving the Bedpan
  Procedure 73 Giving and Receiving the Urinal
  Procedure 74 Assisting with Use of the Bedside Commode

UNIT SUMMARY

There are several measures that you can take to add to the general comfort of the patient. These measures include:
- Caring for the patient's teeth and hair.
- Shaving the patient.
- Giving backrubs to soothe and stimulate.
- Meeting elimination needs promptly and providing privacy.

Early morning or AM care:
- Refreshes the patient before breakfast.
- Prepares the patient for the day.

Bedtime or PM care is a similar procedure that is followed in the evening before sleep. It helps he patient to:

■ Relax.

■ Prepare for sleep.

NURSING ASSISTANT ALERT

Action	Benefit
Carry out hygiene measures that patients cannot do for themselves.	Improves patient comfort.
Encourage patients to assist when possible.	Builds self-esteem and supports independence.
Give AM care in a pleasant manner.	Sets a positive tone for the day.
Provide PM care in an unrushed manner.	Helps patients relax and be more inclined to sleep.
Provide privacy.	Contributes to patient's emotional security.
Meet elimination needs promptly.	Reduces patient discomfort. Aids in promoting normal elimination.

ACTIVITIES

Vocabulary Exercise. Find in the word puzzle each term listed and circle it.

```
L E S O R A L H Y G I E N E C
A V H A J P R A I M S G N C D
J Q O K W C L L P F K O A S T
P B S F S E M I B A C K R U B
E X N E T A Q T K D Q P I F R
I F L C K H P O L E O B M K C
D E N T U R E S S D J A I T L
F Y H S P X F I I C A R I E S
O C M R O A N S Q T M H L N H
B W D O R L G T E R B V F E T
A G K P H E B M F E C E S P A
```

1. false teeth
2. massage of the back
3. unpleasant breath
4. care of mouth and teeth
5. dental cavities
6. solid waste

Completion. Complete the following statements in the spaces provided.

7. When out of the mouth, dentures should be stored in a

_____ .

8. Petroleum jelly or glycerine is applied to the lips for

_____ .

9. Dentures should be handled _____ to prevent damage.

10. The denture storage container should be labeled with

_____ .

11 Proper mouth cleaning helps prevent halitosis and dental _____ .

12. A toothbrush should be inserted into the mouth with the bristles in a _____ position.

13. Special oral hygiene solutions commonly used are mouthwash and a mixture of _____ .

14. Solutions are usually applied with _____ .

15. If possible, the patient should be in a _____ position during toothbrushing.

16. To protect dentures during cleaning, always use a gentle stream of _____ water.

17. Using powder during the backrub can result in irritating _____ .

18. A special order is needed to shave the face of an elderly _____ .

19. When shaving a patient's face, the skin should be held _____ .

20. Brushing the hair makes the patient feel better and _____ the scalp.

21. Before breakfast, the patient should be given the opportunity to go to the bathroom or to use the

_____ .

22. Evening care should be given in a _____ , _____ manner.

23. During evening care, be sure to clear the _____ table and adjust the _____ of the bed.

24. Part of AM and PM care includes tightening the _____ and straightening the _____ linen.

25. After PM care, the bed should be in the _____ horizontal position if patient's condition permits.

26. Make sure that all used _____ have been removed from the patient's room.

Brief Answers. Briefly answer the following questions.

27. Why is oral hygiene important?

_____

28. How are dentures kept when the patient is not wearing them?

_____

29. Why are frequent backrubs given to the patient who is not permitted out of bed?

_____

30. Why should assistants keep their fingernails short?

_____

31. Why should the skin be held taut while using the razor?

_____

32. What would you do if you accidentally nicked a patient during the shaving procedure?

_____

33. What solution is used when there are snarls in oily hair?

34. Why should most patients be left alone when using a bedpan, urinal, or commode?

35. Six patients requiring special oral hygiene are those who are:

a. _____   d. _____

b. _____   e. _____

c. _____   f. _____

36. Five times when backrubs are usually given are:

    a. _____

    b. _____

    c. _____

    d. _____

    e. _____

37. List the equipment you would need to give a backrub.

    a. _____

    b. _____

    c. _____

38. Why is mouth care given before the patient has breakfast?

    _____

39. Why is a backrub given to the patient at bedtime?

    _____

40. How do you wake the patient?

    _____

41. Two instances when you would not waken the patient are if she is:

    a. _____

    b. _____

42. Three activities you will carry out as part of bedtime care include:

    a. _____

    b. _____

    c. _____

Identifying Strokes. Using a colored pencil or crayon, draw in the indicated strokes.

43. Soothing   44. Passive   45. Circular

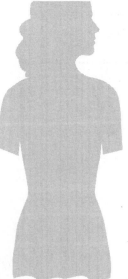
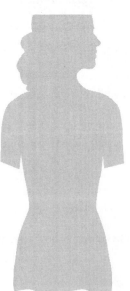
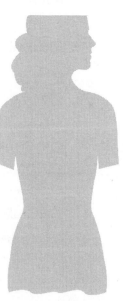

True/False. Mark the following true or false by circling T or F.

46. T   F   Never place a bedpan on the overbed table.

47. T   F   Place the bedpan cover on the bedside stand.

48. T   F   Warm the bedpan by filling with very hot water.

49. T   F   You do not need to cover a used bedpan if the bathroom is close to the patient's room.

50. T   F   A small folded towel can be used to pad a bedpan if the patient is very thin.

51. T   F   If the patient is very heavy, you may need assistance placing him on a bedpan.

52. T   F   The patient's buttocks should rest on the narrow end of the bedpan.

53. T   F   The curtains should be drawn around a patient who is using a bedpan.

54. T   F   Make sure the signal cord is close at hand when the patient is on a bedpan.

55. T   F   Bedpan contents should be noted and documented.

Name the Equipment Enter the name of the equipment pictured in the space provided.

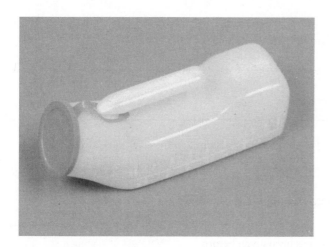

56. _____

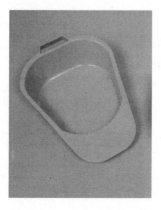

57. _____

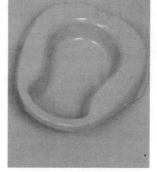

58. _____

Clinical Situations. Briefly describe how a nursing assistant should react to the following situations.

59. You note a pressure area on your patient's hip while giving a backrub.

_____

_____

60. Your patient needs a shave, but he is receiving oxygen and the orders require that the oxygen be administered without interruption. _____

_____

61. Your patient needs to use the bedpan, but cannot lift her buttocks off the bed.

_____

_____

62. You are giving PM care and the patient says he would like to finish the chapter he is reading.

_____

63. Your patient is scheduled for 9 AM surgery and you are assigned to provide AM care to the patient in her room.

_____

64. Your patient is settled for the night and you are ready to leave the room.

_____

RELATING TO THE NURSING PROCESS

Write the step of the nursing process that is related to the nursing assistant action.

Nursing Assistant Action	Nursing Process Step
65. The nursing assistant allows the patient to sleep and omits early AM care because the patient is going to surgery.	_____
66. The nursing assistant makes sure bedtime care has been given before sleep medications are ready.	_____
67. The nursing assistant uses cool water when brushing the dentures for the patient.	_____
68. The nursing assistant reports that the patient's lips are very dry and cracked.	_____
69. The nursing assistant listens carefully when the patient says he doesn't want to put his dentures in because they hurt.	_____
70. The nursing assistant reports and documents the condition of the patient's skin each time she gives back care.	_____

UNIT 25   Nutritional Needs and Diet Modifications

OBJECTIVES

As a result of this unit, you will be able to:

- Spell and define terms.

- Define normal nutrition.

- List types of alternative nutrition.

- List the essential nutrients.

- Name six food groups and list the foods included in each group.

- State the liquids/foods allowed on the five basic facility diets.

- Describe the purposes of the following diets:

- clear liquid

- full liquid

- soft

- light

- State the purposes of therapeutic diets.

- Describe the nursing assistant actions when patients are unable to drink fluids independently.

- Demonstrate the following procedures:

  Procedure 75 Assisting the Patient Who can Feed Self
  Procedure 76 Feeding the Dependent Patient

UNIT SUMMARY

Food is usually taken into the body through the mouth. Sometimes, however, alternative ways of meeting dietary needs must be found. For example:

- Enteral feeding.

- Hyperalimentation.

The nutritional needs are best met when selections are made properly from the six food groups:

- Meat.

- Dairy.

- Vegetables.

- Fruits.

- Breads, cereals, and pastas.

- Fats, oil, and sweets.

Foods for hospital diets are selected from the six food groups. They are prepared in special ways. There are four routine hospital diets:

- House, regular or select
- Liquid, clear
- Liquid, full
- Soft

Many special or therapeutic diets are also prescribed. The patient's dietary intake is based on:
- Personal preference
- Health requirements
- Religious preferences

Fluid intake and output must be carefully balanced for good health:
- Fluids are measured in milliliters (mL) on its equivalent, cubic centimeters (cc).
- Fluids come from and are lost through multiple sources.
- Fluid intake and output must be accurately measured and recorded when ordered.

The assistant helps meet the patient's nutritional needs by:
- Serving trays
- Serving special nourishments
- Providing fresh drinking water
- Assisting patients with feeding
- Feeding patients who are unable to feed themselves

NURSING ASSISTANT ALERT

Action	Benefit
Check diet against patient wrist band.	Ensures patient or proper nutrition.
Present food attractively.	Encourages poor appetites.
Use an unhurried attitude.	Patients improve consumption when not rushed.
Follow orders regarding food or fluid restrictions.	Restrictions are part of the therapy in many conditions.
Measure intake and output carefully.	Findings contribute to accurate evaluation.

ACTIVITIES

Vocabulary Exercise. Complete the puzzle by filling in the missing letters of the words found in this unit. Use the definitions to help you discover these words.

1. N _ _ _ _ _ _ _ _
2. _ _ _ _ U _ _ _ _
3. _ _ _ _ _ _ T _ _ _
4. _ _ _ _ _ _ _ _ R _ _ _ _
5. _ _ _ _ _ _ _ I _ _
6. _ _ _ _ E _ _
7. _ _ N _ _ _ _ _
8. _ _ T _ _ _ _ _
9. _ _ _ S

1. the process by which the body uses food for growth and repair
2. supplies roughage
3. elimination of solid wastes
4. energy foods
5. process of breaking down food into simple substances that can be used for nourishment
6. nutrient used for building and repair
7. inorganic chemical nutrients
8. nutrients necessary for normal metabolism
9. nutrients used to store energy

Completion. Complete the following statements in the spaces provided.

10. The well-nourished person will have a well-developed _____ and body weight appropriate to _____.

11. Hyperalimentation introduces _____ nutrients into a large vein.

12. TPN, which stands for _____ , requires special skill.

13. Carbohydrates and fats are called _____ foods because the body uses them to produce heat and energy.

14. Proteins are composed of _____ acids.

15. Complete proteins contain all the _____ acids that the body _____ manufacture.

16. Following surgery, patients have intake restricted until _____ _____.

17. The first postoperative intake usually permitted is _____ or sips of water.

18. The clear liquid diet does not irritate the bowel or encourage _____ _____.

19. The daily intake of fluid (water) should be _____ glasses.

20. The patient with a fever should be given a (an) _____ diet.

21. The exchange lists are used in preparing a (an) _____ diet.

22. The exchange lists are based on standard _____ measurements.

23. If a patient is on I&O and you serve him nourishments, you must _____ _____.

24. Before serving a tray, be sure to clear away anything that is _____ _____.

25. When feeding the helpless patient, the spoon should be held at a _____ to the patient's mouth.

26. Nutritional supplements are ordered by the physician and have _____ .

True/False. Mark the following true or false by circling T or F.

27. T F   Patients who are unable to swallow without aspiration require alternative nutrition.

28. T F   TPN is a technique that introduces concentrated nutrients into a large vein.

29. T F   Enteral feedings are introduced into smaller veins in the arm.

30. T F   Gastrostomy feedings enter the stomach through a nasogastric tube.

31. T F   Enteral feedings are usually controlled by an automatic device.

32. T F   Oral hygiene may be safely omitted when patients receive enteral feedings, because food doesn't enter the mouth.

33. T F   Nausea or vomiting must be reported immediately to the nurse.

34. T F   The head of the bed should be flat during feedings and remain in that position for half an hour after.

35. T F   Patients must not be permitted to lie on enteral tubes.

36. T F   If tape is causing irritation, the nurse should be informed.

Brief Answers. Briefly answer the following questions.

37. What are the names of three health care facility diets?

    a. _____

    b. _____

    c. _____

38. Why is an unhurried attitude important when feeding a patient?

    _____

39. What is meant by the order to force fluids?

    _____

40. Nutrients may be given by mouth, intravenously, and by two other methods. They are:

    a. _____

    b. _____

41. Three functions of nutrients are:

    a. _____

    b. _____

    c. _____

42. The six basic nutrients are:

    a. _____

    b. _____

    c. _____

    d. _____

    e. _____

    f. _____

43. Four examples of complete proteins are:

    a. _____

    b. _____

    c. _____

    d. _____

44. Four examples of incomplete proteins are:

    a. _____

    b. _____

    c. _____

    d. _____

45. Six minerals needed in our daily diet include:

    a. _____

    b. _____

    c. _____

    d. _____

    e. _____

    f. _____

46. Four functions of vitamins are to:

    a. _____

    b. _____

    c. _____

    d. _____

47. Six vitamins needed by the body are:

    a. _____

    b. _____

    c. _____

    d. _____

    e. _____

    f. _____

48. Name the five "P" foods to be avoided in a low-sodium diet.

    a. _____

    b. _____

    c. _____

    d. _____

    e. _____

49. What are the amounts of average servings?

    a. fruit _____

    b. cooked fruit or vegetable _____

    c. meat _____

    d. pasta/bread_____

50. Intake and output records are kept when specifically ordered for six special circumstances, such as in patients who:

    a. _____

    b. _____

    c. _____

    d. _____

    e. _____

    f. _____

51. Output that must be recorded includes:

    a. _____

    b. _____

    c. _____

    d. _____

    e. _____

    f. _____

52. What does intake include?

    _____

53. What does output include?

    _____

54. In what unit of measurement are intake and output recorded?

    _____

55. For what period of time are intake and output totaled?

    _____

Matching. Identify the type of vitamin.

56. _____   vitamin A   a. water-soluble

57. _____   vitamin B complex   b. fat-soluble

58. _____   vitamin C

59. _____   vitamin D

60. _____   vitamin E

61. _____   vitamin K

Classification. Complete the chart in the spaces provided.

62. Write the names for the six food groups at the top of each column below. Write the names of each of the following foods in the column under the proper food group.

apples	bacon	beef	bread	butter	cereal
cheese	chicken	cottage cheese	fish	flour	honey
ice cream	liver	milk	olive oil	pasta	pears
peas	rice	spinach	yogurt		

_____	_____	_____	_____	_____	_____
Group 1	**Group 2**	**Group 3**	**Group 4**	**Group 5**	**Group 6**
_____	_____	_____	_____	_____	_____
_____	_____	_____	_____	_____	_____
_____	_____	_____	_____	_____	_____
_____	_____	_____	_____	_____	_____
_____	_____	_____	_____	_____	_____

Clinical Situations. Briefly describe how a nursing assistant should react to the following situations.

63. Your patient is on I&O and you picked up the lunch tray. _____

_____

64. You serve a tray to a blind person who is able to feed himself. _____

_____

65. Your patient's chart includes an order to force fluids. _____

_____

66. The patient receiving an IV has 25 mL of fluid left in the bag. _____

_____

_____

67. Your patient is on a strict kosher diet and the tray has a shrimp salad as an entree. _____

_____

Conversions. Convert the following values into milliliters. Show your work.

68. a. 2 (8 oz) cups of coffee _____ _____ mL

b. 1 (6 oz) bowl of soup _____ _____ mL

c. 3 (8 oz) glasses of water _____ _____ mL

d. 2 (4 oz) glasses of ice chips _____ _____ mL

e. 2 (4 oz) dishes of gelatin _____ _____ mL

Completion.

69. Keep a diary of your food intake for 24 hours. Include everything you eat. Then determine if you have achieved an adequate intake of nutrients by answering the questions that follow.

Dietary Chart

Time	Food	Amount

Answer the following questions by entering Yes or No in the space provided.

_____ Did you include two or three servings from the meat group?

_____ Did you include six to eleven servings from the bread, cereal, rice, and pasta group?

_____ Did you include two or more glasses of milk or its equivalent in dairy products?

_____ Did you include at least one serving of a food high in vitamin C.

_____ Did you make sure there was some roughage in your diet?

_____ Did you include three to five servings of the vegetable group?

_____ Are there things in your diet that you think should be eliminated?

70. Complete the food pyramid. Indicate the types of food and number of daily servings.

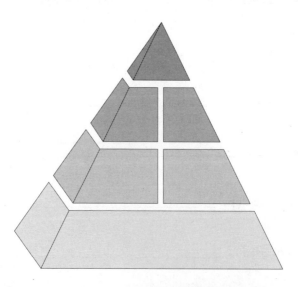

71. Complete an intake and output sheet which reflects the following information. The patient, John Rodriquez, is in Room 404B. During the day he felt fairly well. He drank about 50 mL of water after he brushed his teeth at 0715. He also voided 550 mL of yellow urine. Breakfast arrived and he had a pot of tea (240 mL). Early morning nourishments arrived and he selected and consumed 120 mL of cranberry juice followed by 80 mL of water at lunch (1115) with 120 mL of orange sherbet for dessert. He voided again, 400 mL yellow urine at 1430. During the afternoon he had 240 mL of tea with a visitor. Dinner arrived and he had 180 mL of milk, 180 mL of soup, and 120 mL of gelatin. He asked for a urinal and voided 375 mL of urine. At 2130 he tried to eat some gelatin, approximately 50 mL, and within minutes vomited 400 mL. He continued to feel nauseated and vomited 200 mL at 2315, 150 mL at 2400 and 80 mL at 0230. At 0530 500 mL D/W were started IV. Mr. Rodriquez voided 300 mL at this time. The urine was pink tinged.

WASHINGTON GENERAL HOSPITAL
FLUID INTAKE AND OUTPUT

Name _____   Room _____

Date	Time	Method of Adm.	Intake			Output		
			Solution	Amounts Rec'd	Time	Urine Amount	Others Kind	Amount
Total								

RELATING TO THE NURSING PROCESS

Write the step of the nursing process that is related to the nursing assistant action.

Nursing Assistant Action	Nursing Process Step
72. The nursing assistant carefully checks the patient's identification band against the tray tag.	_____
73. The nursing assistant reports to the nurse that the patient ate only one-third of the soft diet ordered.	_____
74. The nursing assistant documents that the patient refused lunch because he felt nauseated.	_____
75. The nursing assistant carefully records the fluids taken by the patient who has an order for I&O.	_____
76. The nursing assistant checks with the team leader to be sure gelatin should be recorded as fluid intake.	_____
77. The nursing assistant makes a special note during report that her patient is on I&O.	_____

DEVELOPING GREATER INSIGHT

78. Make a statement to the class about the actions you would take if:

    a. Your patient is on I&O and you find a container of milk one-third full when you pick up trays.

    b. Your patient is on I&O and has perspired so much during the night that you had to change the pillowcase and sheet.

79. Try to identify the feelings you might experience if you were an Orthodox Jew and roast pork was served to you.

80. Think through what action you might take while caring for Roman Catholic patient who is to receive Communion at 8 AM and breakfast is served at 7 AM.

81. Working in groups, plan how you would modify the regular diet for an 82-year-old, 110 pound woman who wears dentures.

82. Practice feeding and being fed. Discuss your feelings during the experience.

UNIT 26   Warm and Cold Applications

OBJECTIVES

As a result of this unit, you will be able to:

■ Spell and define terms.

■ List the physical conditions requiring the use of heat and cold.

■ Name types of heat and cold applications.

■ Describe the effects of local cold applications.

■ Describe the effects of local heat applications.

■ List safety concerns related to application of heat and cold.

■ Demonstrate the following procedures:

Procedure 77 Applying and Ice Bag
Procedure 78 Applying a Disposable Cold Pack
Procedure 79 Applying an Aquamatic K-Pad®
Procedure 80 Performing a Warm Soak
Procedure 81 Applying a Warm Moist Compress
Procedure 82 Assisting with Application of a Hypothermia Blanket

UNIT SUMMARY

Treatments with warmth and cold are sometimes performed by nursing assistants. They must be performed with great caution to prevent injury to the patient. The procedures must be performed following the facility policy and be nursing assistant functions as permitted by state law.

These treatments:

■ Require a physician's or registered nurse's order which specifies type, length, and temperature of treatment.

■ Are supervised by a nurse.

■ Must be done in a way that protects the patient against contact with metal, plastic, or rubber.

■ Include applying:

Disposable cold packs.
Aquamatic K-Pads®.
Moist compresses.
Gel packs.

■ Include performing:

Warm foot soaks.
Warm arm soaks.
Cooling sponge baths.

■ Nursing assistants sometimes assist the professional nurse with the application of thermal blankets.

NURSING ASSISTANT ALERT

Action	Benefit
Be sure there is a physician's or registered nurse's order for treatment.	Ensures proper therapy for the correct patient.
Know the reason for and potential response to each technique.	Allows prompt nursing intervention in the event of an untoward reaction.
	Effectiveness of therapy can be reported and evaluated.
Carry out all safety precautions.	Avoids injury and burns.
Expose only necessary parts.	Protects patient privacy. Guards against chilling or discomfort.

ACTIVITIES

Vocabulary Exercise. Complete the crossword puzzle by using the definitions presented.

Down

1. when blood vessels become smaller in diameter
2. excessive blood loss

Across

3. heating mattress
4. immersion of body part in water that is about 105°F.
5. greatly reduced temperature
6. treatment with heat
7. when blood vessels become larger
8. Reusable waterproof canvas container filled with ice cubes.

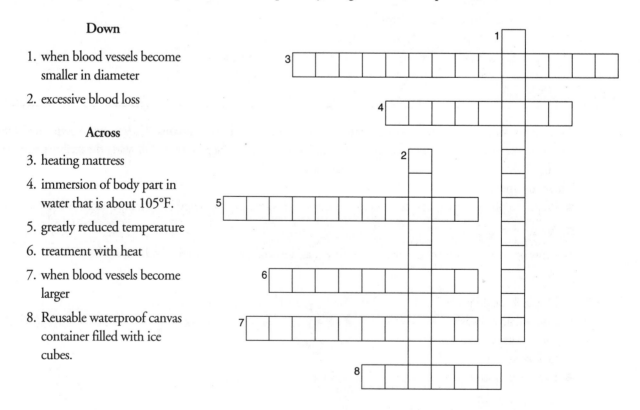

Completion. Complete the following statements in the spaces provided.

9. Two types of hot and cold applications are _____ and _____ .

10. Examples of hot applications are _____ , _____ , and _____ .

11. Examples of cold applications are _____ , _____ , and _____ .

12. When adding water to a warm foot soak, always _____ the feet.

13. An ice bag should be filled _____ .

14. When filling an ice bag, pressing the hand against the flat surface expels the _____ .

15. No application of heat or cold can be given without _____

_____ .

16. The Aquamatic K-Pad® control unit should be filled with _____ .

17. After securing the cap on an Aquamatic K-Pad® control unit, the cap must be loosened _____ turn.

18. Use of a hyperthermia blanket is a _____ nursing responsibility.

19. A thermal mattress used to reduce body temperature is known as a _____

_____ .

20. Applications of cold to a sprained ankle can reduce _____ and numb sensation of

_____ .

21. Warm application causes blood vessels to _____ .

_____ .

22. When using plastic containers to apply heat, care must be taken that the patient's skin does not touch the _____ .

23. Heat should not be applied to the head because it can cause _____ .

24. If there is a question of appendicitis, _____ should not be applied to the abdomen.

25. Check all areas to which cold is applied for _____ and _____ .

26. Before fastening the cap of an ice bag securely, all _____ should be expelled.

27. The metal cap of an ice bag should always be positioned _____ from the patient.

28. To activate a commercial cold pack, _____ or squeeze the pack.

29. Patients should never be allowed to _____ on an Aquamatic K-Pad® .

30. The prescribed temperature for an arm or foot soak is about _____ °F.

31. For accuracy, the temperature of all warm or cold treatments should be checked with a _____ .

32. An _____ or syringe may be used to apply additional solution to keep moist treatments moist.

33. Before applying a moist compress, always remove _____ .

34. The Aquamatic K-Pad® cord must be plugged into an _____ for the unit to operate.

35. Always check a warm water bottle for _____ before applying.

36. A warm water bottle should always be _____ before application.

37. Aquamatic K-Pads® are _____ used in a health care facility.

38. Four reasons for applying heat or cold are to:

    a. _____

    b. _____

    c. _____

    d. _____

39. Three ways to apply dry cold are by:

    a. _____

    b. _____

    c. _____

40. Three ways moist cold is applied are by:

    a. _____

    b. _____

    c. _____

41. Warm and cold applications must be used with special caution with certain patients. Four such patients are those who are:

    a. _____

    b. _____

    c. _____

    d. _____

42. List the information needed to document a warm or cold treatment.

    a. _____

    b. _____

    c. _____

    d. _____

    e. _____

43. List the equipment needed for a warm foot soak.

    a. _____

    b. _____

    c. _____

    d. _____

    e. _____

    f. _____

    g. _____

True/False. Mark the following statements relating to a warm arm soak true or false by circling T or F.

44. T   F   When doing a warm arm soak, keep the bed flat.

45. T   F   The patient should be positioned to the far side of the bed opposite the arm to be soaked.

46. T   F   The temperature of the water should be checked every 30 minutes.

47. T   F   The arm soak basin should be two-thirds filled with water.

48. T   F   The temperature of the water is usually 115°F.

49. T   F   Protect bedding with plastic and a towel during the soaking.

50. T   F   The procedure is so routine it need not be documented.

51. T   F   Warm water may be added during the soak to maintain the temperature.

52. T   F   Beginning procedure actions should be carried out.

53. T   F   Equipment should be stored under the bed until needed again.

Clinical Situations. Briefly describe how a nursing assistant should react to the following situations.

54. You found the cover of the Aquamatic K-Pad® unit screwed on tightly. _____

_____

55. You found an ice bag without a cloth cover being used on a patient. _____

_____

_____

56. The patient receiving a cold treatment complained of numbness in the part being treated.

_____

RELATING TO THE NURSING PROCESS

Write the step of the nursing process that is related to the nursing assistant action.

Nursing Assistant Action	Nursing Process Step
57. The nursing assistant is instructed to apply an ice bag to the patient's arm. She is unsure of how long to leave it in place and asks the nurse.	_____
58. The nursing assistant covers the ice bag with a towel so that the bag is not directly against a patient's skin.	_____
59. The nursing assistant reports the patient's reaction to the placement of a warm water bag.	_____
60. The nursing assistant uses tape to secure the Aquamatic K-Pad® in place over the patient's leg.	_____

DEVELOPING GREATER INSIGHT

61. Explain why air should be removed from an ice bag before application.

62. Describe the danger of not removing the patient's leg before adding hot water to a foot soak.

63. Assist the professional nurse with a hypothermia blanket. Think of the reasons this treatment might be administered.

64. Discuss with classmates the dangers of improperly applied treatments of heat and cold.

UNIT 27   Assisting with the Physical Examination

OBJECTIVES

As a result of this unit, you will be able to:
- Spell and define terms.
- Describe the responsibilities of the nursing assistant during the physical assessment.
- Name the positions for the various physical examinations.
- Drape patient for the various positions.
- Name the basic instruments necessary for physical examinations.
- Demonstrate the following procedure:

  Procedure 83 Assisting with a Physical Examination

UNIT SUMMARY

Another member of the staff must be present during a physical examination. The nursing assistant may assist the physician during the physical examination and as the nurse performs a nursing assessment. You do this successfully when you:
- Provide privacy while the patient's history is discussed.
- Are ready to assist during the examination and to provide proper lighting.
- Avoid overexposing the patient as you adjust the drapes.
- Remember that most patients feel uneasy about physical examinations. Be reassuring.
- Drape and position patients safely while maintaining proper body mechanics.
- Know and prepare the proper equipment for the examination.
- Assist patients during the examination and after the examination is completed.
- Properly clean up the room and equipment after the examination is completed.

NURSING ASSISTANT ALERT

Action	Benefit
Position patients for optimum comfort, safety and privacy.	Prevents injury. Reduces anxiety. Facilitates the examination.
Have all necessary equipment and supplies ready.	Saves time, reduces patient stress.
Stay beside and assist patient during position changes.	Provides support and prevents injury.

ACTIVITIES

Vocabulary Exercise. Each line has four different spellings of a word. Circle the correctly spelled word.

1. litotomy   lithotomy   lythotomy   lithotome

2. percussun   percussion   percusion   pacussion

3. autoscope   otascop   otoscope   otascope

4. speculum   specalum   spiculum   specolom

5. opthalomoscope   ophthalmoscope   ophtalmoscope   ophtholmascope

Definitions. Define the following words.

6. dorsal recumbent _____

7. drape _____

8. flexed _____

9. percussion hammer_____

10. ophthalmoscope _____

11. otoscope _____

12. speculum _____

Completion. Complete the following statements in the spaces provided.

13. When in the lithotomy position, the knees are _____.

14. When in the dorsal recumbent position, the patient lies on his _____.

15. When in the knee-chest position, the patient should never be _____.

16. When in the prone position, the patient lies on his _____.

17. When in Sims' position, the patient lies on his _____ side.

18. The basic examination position is _____.

19. The position used for a pelvic examination is _____.

20. The position sometimes used for a rectal examination is the _____.

21. Patients are usually draped in cloth or paper _____.

22. However the draping is done, it is important that the patient _____ covered.

23. The most common position for head and neck examination is _____.

24. Name the positions pictured.

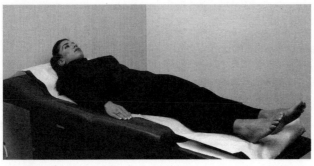

a. _____

b. _____

c. _____

d. _____

Brief Answers. Briefly explain each of the following.

25. The role of the nursing assistant during a physical examination

_____

_____

26. How the physical examination helps the physician _____

_____

_____

_____

27. List the equipment you will set up for a pelvic examination.

a. _____   f. _____

b. _____   g. _____

c. _____   h. _____

d. _____   i. _____

e. _____

28. Name the instruments and equipment in a physical examination and explain its use.

a. _____   f. _____

b. _____   g. _____

c. _____   h. _____

d. _____   i. _____

e. _____

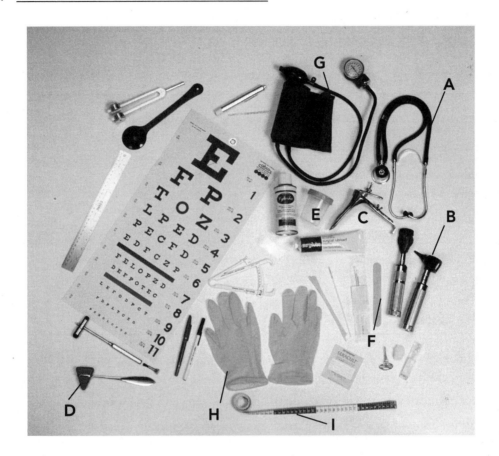

Clinical Situations. Briefly describe how a nursing assistant should react to the following situations.

29. The patient seems very nervous before a physical examination. _____

_____

30. The physician wants to do a pelvic examination. _____

_____

_____

31. The nurse wants to examine the patient's throat and chest. _____

_____

True/False. Mark the following true or false by circling T or F.

32. T   F   A physical examination helps the physician establish a diagnosis.

33. T   F   The nursing assistant examines the patient to make a nursing diagnosis.

34. T   F   The nursing assistant should expose only the part being examined.

35. T   F   The nursing assistant doesn't need to know how to operate the examination table, because the physician will perform this task.

36. T   F   When in the horizontal recumbent position, the patient is placed on her abdomen.

37. T   F   The semi-Fowler's position is often used when the head and neck are to be examined.

38. T   F   Patients should void before the pelvic examination.

39. T   F   A Pap smear is usually taken with the patient in the semi-Fowler's position.

40. T   F   Before examination begins, privacy must be provided.

41. T   F   The nursing assistant should try to anticipate the examiner's needs.

RELATING TO THE NURSING PROCESS

Write the step of the nursing process that is related to the nursing assistant action.

Nursing Assistant Action	Nursing Process Step
42. The nursing assistant helps the patient assume the dorsal lithotomy position for a pelvic examination.	_____
43. The nursing assistant records information as the physician or nurse carries out the examination.	_____
44. The nursing assistant measures the patient's height and weight and passes instruments during the physical examination.	_____

DEVELOPING GREATER INSIGHT

45. Try positioning yourself in the knee-chest and lithotomy positions. Think carefully of how you feel. What might be done to increase your feelings of privacy and security?

46. Ask your instructor to let you try on a hospital or examination gown. Did you feel covered?

47. Examine the instruments used for the physical examination. Describe for classmates their purposes.

UNIT 28   The Surgical Patient

OBJECTIVES

As a result of this unit, you will be able to:

- Spell and define terms.

- Describe the concerns of patients who are about to have surgery.

- List the various types of anesthesia.

- Shave the operative area.

- Prepare the patient's unit for the patient's return from the operating room.

- Prepare a recovery bed.

- Demonstrate the following procedures:

    Procedure 84 Shaving the Operative Area
    Procedure 85 Assisting Patient to Deep Breathe and Cough
    Procedure 86 Performing Postoperative Leg Exercises
    Procedure 87 Applying Elasticized Stockings
    Procedure 88 Applying Elastic Bandage
    Procedure 89 Assisting Patient to Dangle

UNIT SUMMARY

The surgical patient requires continuous care before, during, and after surgery. The nursing assistant helps in preoperative and postoperative care.

Nursing assistant responsibilities in the preoperative period include:

- Preparing the operative site.

- Readying the patient on the morning of surgery.

- Helping in the transfer of the patient to and from the stretcher.

- Providing emotion support.

Nursing assistant responsibilities during the operative period include:

- Preparing a surgical (postoperative) bed.

- Securing equipment needed for the postoperative period.

Nursing assistant responsibilities in the postoperative period include:

- Assisting in the transfer from stretcher to bed.

- Carefully observing and reporting.

- Assisting the patient with postoperative exercises, including:

    Position changes.
    Leg exercises.
    Respiratory exercises.

- Applying elasticized stockings.
- Assisting in dangling and initial ambulation
- Using standard precautions any time that contact with blood, body fluids, secretions, excretions, mucous membranes, or nonintact skin is likely.

NURSING ASSISTANT ALERT

Action	Benefit
Provide emotional support by being calm, efficient, and a willing listener.	Builds patient confidence and helps reduce fears.
Carry out pre- and postoperative orders carefully.	Reduces the likelihood of postoperative complications.
Assemble necessary equipment and conscientiously prepare the patient's room for his return from surgery.	Appropriate care can be immediately given as needed. Time is not wasted.
Observe the patient closely as postoperative exercise and ambulation are attempted. Be prepared to assist.	Avoids patient injury.
Report observations accurately and promptly.	Proper nursing interventions may be employed that promote recovery.

ACTIVITIES

Vocabulary Exercise. Complete the puzzle by filling in the missing letters of words found in this unit. Use the definitions to help you discover these words.

1. _ _ _ _ _ _ _ S _ _   1. artificial body part
2. _ _ _ U _ _ _ _ _ _   2. walking
3. _ _ R _ _ _ _   3. dizziness
4. _ _ _ G _ _ _ _ _   4. hiccup
5. _ _ _ _ _ I _ _   5. sitting with feet over bed edge
6.   C   6.
7. _ _ _ _ _ _ _ A _ _ _   7. collapse of lung tissue
8. _ _ _ _ L _ _ _ _ _   8. removes hair

Matching. Match the word on the right with the statements on the left.

9. ____   hospital-acquired   a. embolus

10. ____   the period following surgery   b. dyspnea

11. ____   drawing foreign material into the lungs   c. pallor

12. ____   lack of adequate oxygen supply   d. nosocomial

13. ____   loss of feeling or sensation   e. thrombus

14. ____   stationary blood clot   f. vertigo

15. ____   dizziness   g. thrombophlebitis

16. ____   less than normal skin color   h. postoperative

17. ____   difficulty breathing   i. hypoxia

18. ____   moving blood clot   j. aspiration

                                                         k. anesthesia

Completion. Complete the following statements in the spaces provided.

19. The three phases of care required by the surgical patient are:

    a. _____

    b. _____

    c. _____

20. The purpose of anesthesia is _____.

21. Gaseous anesthetics are _____.

22. When patients have general anesthesia, they are apt to _____ postoperatively.

23. Gaseous anesthetics keep the patient _____ during surgery.

24. During a local anesthetic, the patient may remain _____ during surgery.

25. When a spinal anesthetic is given, all sensations _____ the level of the injection are _____ .

26. Intravenous anesthetics make the patient fall asleep _____.

27. Seven duties the nursing assistant may be assigned in regard to the preoperative patient are:

    a. _____

    b. _____

    c. _____

    d. _____

    e. _____

    f. _____

    g. _____

28. Equipment left on the bedside table after the recovery bed is made includes:

_____

29. When a patient vomits, his head should be _____ to prevent _____ .

30. Spinal anesthesia is often given for abdominal surgery because it produces good _____.

31. Patient questions should be referred to the _____.

32. The patient's position should be changed every _____ hours following surgery.

33. You should always check the patient's _____ frequently as the patient dangles or ambulates for the first time.

34. Binders that are ordered postoperatively must be:

    a. _____

    b. _____

    c. _____

35. Elasticized stockings or Ace bandages are applied postoperatively to help support the _____ of the legs.

36. Postoperative leg exercises should be performed _____ times every _____ hours.

Complete the following statements regarding postoperative discomfort in the spaces provided.

37. The patient complains of thirst. You should give special _____ care and check for signs of _____ .

38. The patient has singultus. You should support the _____ area.

39. The patient complains of pain. You should report the _____ , _____ , and _____ of pain.

40. The patient's abdomen is distended. You should encourage increased _____ .

41. The patient has urinary retention. You should monitor _____ carefully.

42. The patient is hemorrhaging. You should keep the patient quiet and check _____ .

43. The patient may be going into shock. You suspect this because there is a fall in _____ , the pulse is _____ , the skin is _____ , and its color is pale.

44. The patient is suffering from hypoxia. You should _____ position and monitor oxygen if ordered.

45. The patient has suffered wound disruption. You should keep the patient _____ and _____ the incision area.

46. If a depilatory is used before surgery to remove hair, the nursing assistant should _____ .

47. If the skin area to which a depilatory has been applied becomes reddened, the nursing assistant should _____ .

48. If an electric clipper is used to prepare the operative area, the heads should be _____ or _____ .

Surgical Prep Areas. Shade in the surgical prep areas that are to be shaved before surgery with colored pencil or crayon as indicated.

49. a. Abdominal surgery

    b. breast surgery—anterior

    c. breast surgery—posterior

    d. back surgery

    e. kidney surgery

    f. vaginal, rectal, and perineal surgery

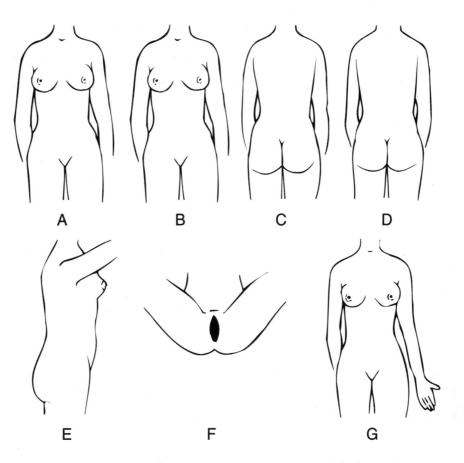

A   B   C   D

E   F   G

Brief Answers. Answer the following questions.

50. What is needed for pain sensations to be realized?

   a. _____

   b. _____

   c. _____

51. What information is taught to the patient before surgery?

   a. _____

   b. _____

   c. _____

52. What can the nursing assistant do to build patient confidence?

   a. _____

   b. _____

   c. _____

   d. _____

   e. _____

53. Why must nosocomial infections be prevented?

   a. _____

   b. _____

   c. _____

54. What actions should you take before the final preoperative medication is given?

  a. _____

  b. _____

  c. _____

  d. _____

  e. _____

  f. _____

  g. _____

55. What actions should you take after the medication is given?

  a. _____

  b. _____

  c. _____

  d. _____

  e. _____

56. What actions would you take while the patient is in the operating room?

  a. _____

  b. _____

  c. _____

57. What actions should be taken when the patient returns from surgery?

  a. _____

  b. _____

  c. _____

  d. _____

  e. _____

58. What special precautions should be taken when there are drainage tubes in place?

  a. _____

  b. _____

  c. _____

  d. _____

  e. _____

  f. _____

  g. _____

  h. _____

59. Examine the surgical checklist below. List the articles that are direct nursing assistant responsibilities.

  a. _____   d. _____

  b. _____   e. _____

  c. _____   f. _____

1. Admission sheet
2. Surgical consent
3. Sterilization consent (if necessary)
4. Consultation sheet (if necessary)
5. History and physical
6. Lab reports (pregnancy tests also if necessary)
7. Surgery prep done and charted, if required
8. Latest TPR and blood pressure charted
9. Preoperative medication has been given and charted (if required)
10. Name tape on patient
11. Fingernail polish and makeup removed
12. Metallic objects removed (rings may be taped)
13. Dentures removed
14. Other prostheses removed (such as artificial limb or eye)
15. Bath blanket and head cap in place
16. Bed in high position and side rails up after preop medication is given
17. Patient has voided

Clinical Situations.   Briefly describe how a nursing assistant should react to the following situations.

60. You are assigned to do a pubic prep and your patient's pubic hair is very long. _____

_____

61. You are assisting a patient with initial ambulation, and the patient faints. _____

_____

62 You find that the anti-embolism stockings your patient is wearing are wrinkled and have slipped down his leg.

_____

_____

63. Your postoperative patient's blood pressure has dropped and her pulse is rapid and weak. Her skin is cold and moist. _____

_____

64. Your postoperative patient is anxious, has a feeling of heaviness in his chest, and is cyanotic. _____

_____

RELATING TO THE NURSING PROCESS

Write the step of the nursing process that is related to the nursing assistant action.

Nursing Assistant Action   **Nursing Process Step**

65. The nursing assistant listens to and reports the patient's concerns about scheduled
    surgery to the nurse.   _____

66. The nursing assistant helps the patient bathe or shower with surgical soap.   _____

67. The nursing assistant checks with the nurse to determine the specific area to be
    shaved for surgery.   _____

68. Unattached hairs following shaving are removed by the nursing assistant by
    gently pressing the sticky side of surgical tape against them.   _____

69. The nursing assistant makes sure there are no wrinkles in elasticized stockings
    once they are applied.   _____

70. The nursing assistant finds the patient's pulse rate has increased more than 10 bpm after
    initial standing. The nursing assistant returns the patient to bed and reports to the nurse. _____

DEVELOPING GREATER INSIGHT

73. Discuss ways you can assist a patient to support himself when he tries to cough and deep breathe following
    surgery.

74. Discuss ways you can contribute to the prevention of nosocomial infections.

75. With so many people having short-term surgery today, your contact with surgery patients may be limited. Think
    about ways you can make these contacts the most beneficial to the patient.

UNIT 29 Caring for the Emotionally Stressed Patient

OBJECTIVES

As a result of this unit, you will be able to:

- Spell and define terms.

- Define mental health.

- Explain the interrelatedness of physical and mental health.

- Understand mental health as a process of adaptations.

- Identify commonly used defense mechanisms.

- Describe ways to help patients cope with stressful situations.

- Identify the signs and symptoms of maladaptive behaviors that should be documented and reported.

- List nursing assistant measures in providing care for patients with adaptive and maladaptive reactions.

UNIT SUMMARY

Mental and physical health are interrelated. They influence the individual's ability to cope with his life within the framework of society.

Mental health is maintained through the use of different coping mechanisms such as:

- Repression.

- Suppression.

- Projection.

- Denial.

- Reaction formation.

- Displacement.

- Identification.

- Compensation.

- Conversion.

- Undoing.

Failure of coping mechanisms leads to maladaptive behaviors. These include:

- Excessive demands.

- Alcoholism.

- Depression.

- Disorientation.

- Agitation.

- Paranoia.

- Suicide attempts.

The nursing assistant has specific responsibilities when caring for patients exhibiting maladaptive behaviors. These include:
- Observing and objectively reporting behaviors.
- Ensuring patient safety.
- Intervening in behaviors as directed by the care plan.

NURSING ASSISTANT ALERT

Action	Benefit
Observe and objectively report patient behaviors.	Ensures correct evaluation.
Closely supervisor activities.	Prevents patient injury.
Use consistency in your approach.	Helps patients reorient. Lessens the degree of confusion. Contributes to the patient's sense of security.
Be vigilant in recognizing potentially unsafe situations.	Allows early interventions that reduce the likelihood of injury to patients or staff.

ACTIVITIES

Vocabulary Exercise. Put a circle around the words as indicated and then give an example of each.

1. Locate nine common defense mechanisms or adaptive behaviors. Use the circled letters to get you started.

```
R E P R E S S I O N H E L F J C K E B
D K A I P R C U G Q T B O A R R P H O
A O V C F O I D I S P L A C E M E N T
E H L O T R D R K S B H P E W L S I U
P W C V K I F A P I U A R Z G B U D N
T B R H B I O P L C O H R D T O H E D
O Q E W O C O N V E R S I O N E W N O
U H T G Z O S J B Q G F C P S D D T I
B U A L S M I D P F H W I A H E H I N
L R K C P P U K J I O B R F L N G O G
O Z B S H E A K S U P R E S S I O N K
D S G F P N E F L G E W M J G A O R B
P A L I O S H K D J Z G P A R L G E P
C R A F B A J L A P C A R H T O H I A
S H F A N T A S Y E H S G B E I D L P
I R J K I I E G Q I C O J G I P O K H
E Z B L P O H F P R O J E C T I O N R
M F I E Q N I J G R A R G K A P E O C
```

a. _____

_____

b. _____

_____

c. _____

_____

d. _____

_____

e. _____

_____

f. _____

_____

g. _____

_____

h. _____

_____

i. _____

_____

Completion. Complete the following statements in the spaces provided.

2. Mental health means exhibiting behaviors that reflect a person's _____ to the multiple stress of life.

3. A situation that makes a person anxious about his well-being is called a _____

_____.

4. Poor mental health is demonstrated by _____.

5. Physical and mental health are _____.

6. A word used to mean handling stress is _____ with stress.

7. People use _____ mechanisms to protect their self-esteem.

8. Demanding patients are usually only expressing their own _____.

9. Some people turn to alcohol as a means of _____

_____.

10. Alcohol _____ brain activity.

11. Alcohol is a drug that mixes _____ with other drugs.

12. Older alcoholics have a _____ chance of recovery.

13. The best approach to the disoriented patient is one that is _____ and _____.

14. Agitation is defined as inappropriate vocal or _____ activity due to causes other than confusion or need.

15. The patient who is disoriented may benefit from _____ orientation.

16. An extreme maladaptive response in which the person feels everyone is against him is called _____.

17. The nursing assistant must be sensitive to non_____ clues to the sources of a patient's stress.

18. It is important that the patient who is under stress feels that the nursing assistant is _____ and will respect privacy and feelings.

19. Be supportive of the person's own _____ to overcome the stress.

20. Patients often show their frustrations by being very _____ .

True/False. Mark the following true or false by circling T or F.

21. T F You can help patients cope with stress by being a good listener.

22. T F You should try to make patients see situations from your point of view.

23. T F If you know the patient is wrong, it is all right to argue the point.

24. T F It is permissible for the intoxicated person to smoke unsupervised.

25. T F Disorientation and depression may be associated with both physical and mental disorders.

26. T F The most common functional disorder in the geriatric age group is depression.

27. T F Some properly used drugs can cause a person to feel depressed.

28. T F A proper approach to the depressed patient is to let him know how sorry you feel for him.

29. T F The person who threatens suicide never attempts it.

30. T F An elderly person who has just lost a spouse is a risk for suicide.

31. T F The suicidal patient needs help in restoring his feelings of self-esteem.

32. T F Agitation is a significant problem for the elderly, their families, and the nursing staff.

33. T F The patient who is agitated has a prolonged attention span.

34. T F Constipation and dehydration can contribute to agitation.

35. T F   One way to help the depressed patient is to reinforce his self-concept as a valued member of society.

36. T F   The person who is depressed feels better if you express pity for him.

37. T F   The disoriented person may show disorientation to time, person, or place.

38. T F   Labeling a behavior implies passing judgment.

39. T F   Speaking to others in the same way the supervisor speaks to you is a form of compensation.

Brief Answers. Briefly answer the following questions.

40. List five common life stresses.

   a. _____

   b. _____

   c. _____

   d. _____

   e. _____

41. Explain each of the following defense mechanisms.

   a. projection _____

   _____

   b. denial _____

   _____

   c. identification _____

   _____

   d. fantasy _____

   _____

   e. compensation _____

   _____

42. List four ways to successfully deal with a demanding patient.

   a. _____

   b. _____

   c. _____

   d. _____

43. List five ways a nursing assistant can work with an alcoholic patient.

   a. _____

   b. _____

   c. _____

   d. _____

   e. _____

44. List five signs and symptoms you may note that would indicate that the patient is depressed.

   a. _____

   b. _____

   c. _____

d. _____

e. _____

45. List eight signs and symptoms that indicate disorientation.

a. _____

b. _____

c. _____

d. _____

e. _____

f. _____

g. _____

h. _____

46. List six ways you can help a disoriented patient be better oriented to reality.

a. _____

b. _____

c. _____

d. _____

e. _____

f. _____

Clinical Situations.   Briefly describe how a nursing assistant should react to the following situations.

47. Mrs. Sears has trouble sleeping, seems lethargic, and frequently dabs tears from her eyes.

a. _____

b. _____

c. _____

48. Mr. Osborn is recovering from a head injury sustained in a fall downstairs. He insists that the patient in the next room is his daughter and tries to see her.

a. _____

b. _____

c. _____

d. _____

49. Mrs. Bell is pacing in the corridor. She repeatedly asks the same question of the staff. She sometime bites and spits at others. Explain factors that will contribute to her agitation.

a. _____

b. _____

c. _____

d. _____

e. _____

f. _____

g. _____

h. _____

RELATING TO THE NURSING PROCESS

Write the step of the nursing process that is related to the nursing assistant action.

Nursing Assistant Action   **Nursing Process Step**

50. The nursing assistant listens but doesn't argue even though the patient is wrong in his belief.

_____

51. The nursing assistant reports the patient's use of profanity without "labeling" his behavior.

_____

52. The nurse observes the way the patient says words and the body language he uses at the time.

_____

53. The nursing assistant reports to the nurse about ways she has found to help the patient deal with stress.

_____

54. The nursing assistant acts in a positive way when a patient is depressed.

_____

55. The nursing assistant reports that the patient is experiencing apathy and crying spells.

_____

56. The nursing assistant gives instructions slowly and clearly in simple words to a disoriented person.

_____

DEVELOPING GREATER INSIGHT

57. Complete the chart to demonstrate your understanding of the concept of how people cope with stress. Discuss this with your classmates.

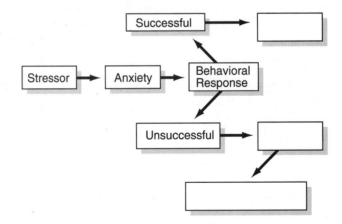

Think carefully about your own coping mechanisms for stress. Could you find more appropriate ways of dealing with stress?

58. Look around your facility or clinical area. Try to identify anything that may be a safety hazard for a disoriented person.

59. Role play with classmates the proper way to manage an agitated patient. Have one student act as the patient.

60. Think about your relationships with your teacher and classmates. Can you identify any situation in which you used one of the defense mechanisms described in this lesson.

61. Discuss with the class ways you personally have found that help reduce stress.

UNIT 30 Death and Dying

OBJECTIVES

As a result of this unit, you will be able to:

- Spell and define terms.

- Describe how different people handle the process of death and dying.

- List the signs of approaching death.

- Describe the nursing assistant's responsibilities for providing supportive care.

- Describe the spiritual preparations for death practiced by various religious denominations.

- Describe the hospice philosophy and method of care.

- Demonstrate the following procedure:

  Procedure 90 Giving Postmortem Care.

UNIT SUMMARY

- Assisting with terminal and postmortem care is a difficult but essential part of nursing duties. It requires a high degree of sensitivity, understanding, and tact.

- Both the patient and the family require support during this trying period.

- Care must be taken to provide for the individual religious preferences and practices of the patient and the family.

- The procedure for postmortem care must be carried out with efficiency and respect.

NURSING ASSISTANT ALERT

Action	Benefit
Recognize that the stages of grief are experienced by patient and family.	Allows staff to provide essential emotional support.
Remember that people react to a terminal diagnosis in a variety of ways.	Permits nursing care to be individualized.
Identify the signs of impending death.	Allows proper nursing care interventions to be carried out.
Treat the body with the same respect as the living patient.	Maintains dignity and respect.

ACTIVITIES

Vocabulary Exercise. Each line has four different spellings of a word. Circle the correctly spelled word.

1. critical	cretical	critecal	creticale
2. posmortum	postmartem	postmortem	postmortom
3. hopice	hopise	hospise	hospice
4. terminale	terminal	termanel	termanal
5. danial	deniel	denial	deniale
6. morabund	moribund	moreband	moribond
7. annointing	anointing	annointen	anontin
8. awtopsie	awtopsy	autopse	autopsy
9. bargaining	bargenan	bargainin	bergaining
10. rigor mortis	rigor mortus	riger mortis	regor mortos

Completion. Complete the statements in the spaces provided.

11. When the patient's condition is critical, the _____ places the patient's name on the critical list.

12. Sacrament of the Sick is requested for the patient of _____ belief.

13. Hospice care is based on the philosophy that death is a _____ process.

14. Hospice care is provided for people with a life expectancy of _____.

15. Hospice care is provided by _____ who work with the patient and the family.

16. As death approaches, body functions _____.

17. The last sense lost is the sense of _____ .

18. As death approaches, the pulse becomes _____ and progressively _____ .

19. The time of death is determined by the _____.

20. Under no circumstances should the _____ inform the family of the patient's death.

21. As a nursing assistant, you have a unique opportunity to be a source of _____ and _____ to the dying patient and the family.

22. During the dying period, you must provide the family and patient with _____.

23. The nursing assistant must realize that dying is a _____ each person must make _____ .

True/False. Mark the following true or false by circling T or F.

24. T F A patient goes through each stage in a sequential order.

25. T F Once he or she has moved on to another stage, the patient never returns to the former stage.

26. T F All patients go through each stage of grieving at the same rate.

27. T F The nursing assistant must have an understanding attitude during each stage.

28. T F The family members may go through the same five stages.

29. T F The nursing assistant should reflect the patient's statements during the stage of denial.

30. T F If the patient seems depressed, it is best to leave him alone to work it out himself.

31. T F It may not be assumed that because the patient is in the stage of acceptance, he has no fear.

32. T   F   The stage of depression is often filled with expression of regrets.

33. T   F   The patient who has reached the stage of acceptance may try to assist those around him to deal with his death.

34. T   F   The Patient Self-Determination Act goes into effect as soon as a patient is admitted to a health care facility.

35. T   F   Supportive care for terminally ill patients does not include life-sustaining treatments.

Brief Answers.   Briefly answer the following questions in the spaces provided.

36. Write the five stages of grief as outlined by E. Kübler-Ross.

   a. _____

   b. _____

   c. _____

   d. _____

   e. _____

37. What are the goals of hospice programs?

   a. _____

   b. _____

   c. _____

38. As a member of the hospice team, how can you promote the hospice policy?

   a. _____

   b. _____

   c. _____

   d. _____

39. What are five moribund changes?

   a. _____

   b. _____

   c. _____

   d. _____

   e. _____

40. What items would you expect to find in a morgue kit?

   a. _____

   b. _____

   c. _____

   d. _____

   e. _____

41. What should you do before moving the body to the morgue, to prevent upsetting other patients?

   _____

   _____

42. Why is the use of standard precautions necessary when performing postmortem care?

_____

_____

Clinical Situations.   Briefly describe how a nursing assistant should react to the following situations.

43. Your terminal patient, who had been crying earlier, suddenly appears cheerful and talks about a trip he is planning for next year.

_____

_____

44. The patient expresses a desire to see his clergy.

_____

45. The physician has pronounced the patient deceased and you are to prepare the patient for the return of the family.

a. _____

b. _____

c. _____

d. _____

e. _____

46. The patient has an order for supportive care only. Explain the care this includes:

a. _____

b. _____

c. _____

d. _____

47. The patient has both a living will and a durable power of attorney. Write the name of the document that assigns responsibility for handling the patient's personal affairs and making health care decisions for the patient.

_____

48. For patients with no-code orders, state how this order influences care if the patients experience respiratory and cardiac arrest.

_____

RELATING TO THE NURSING PROCESS

Write the step of the nursing process that is related to the nursing assistant action.

Nursing Assistant Action	Nursing Process Step
49. The nursing assistant promptly reports complaints of pain by the terminally ill patient to the nurse.	_____
50. During the postmortem period, the nursing assistant cares for the body with dignity.	_____
51. The nursing assistant checks the dying patient frequently.	_____
52. The nursing assistant offers quiet support to the family of the dying patient by listening.	_____

DEVELOPING GREATER INSIGHT

53. Share with classmates any special rituals or practices that your family carries out when someone dies.

54. Invite members of different faiths to share some of their experiences with dying people.

55. Invite a nursing assistant or nurse who works in a hospice to come and share some of his or her experiences with the class.

56. Think how you might feel if you were giving care to a patient who is terminally ill and has an order for supportive care only.

UNIT 31   Care of the Elderly and Chronically Ill

OBJECTIVES

As a result of this unit, you will be able to:

- Spell and define terms.
- List the federal requirements for nursing assistants working in long-term care facilities.
- Identify the expected changes of aging.
- List the actions a nursing assistant can take to prevent infections in the long-term care facility.
- Recognize unsafe conditions in the long-term care facility.
- Describe actions to use when working with residents who have dementia.

UNIT SUMMARY

The person being cared for in the long-term health care facility is:

- Usually a mature adult.
- Often elderly.
- Frequently afflicted with chronic and/or debilitating conditions.

Adult life spans a period of 50 years or more and is divided into:

- Early adulthood   20–40 years
- Middle adulthood   40–65 years
- Late adulthood   65–75 years
- Old age   75 years and over

Basic care will be provided using the same techniques employed in the acute setting. Adaptations must be made because of the greater dependency of this group of residents. Physical changes occur in each body system as aging progresses.

It is important for the nursing assistant to remember that each person is a unique individual and must be treated with respect and dignity.

Adjustments to the aging process must be made on a physical and emotional level. The nursing assistant can be a valuable source of caring and support. Special care needs have to be met in the following areas:

- Promoting residents' rights.
- Caring for personal hygiene.
- Meeting dietary requirements.
- Ensuring adequate exercise.
- Caring for elimination.
- Providing recreational needs.
- Supporting emotional adjustments.
- Orienting to reality.

- Providing a safe environment
- Providing opportunities for social interactions
- Preventing infections

NURSING ASSISTANT ALERT

Action	Benefit
Familiarize yourself with the usual signs of aging.	Forms a baseline of comparison for abnormal findings.
Avoid stereotypes.	Encourages people to be seen as individuals.
Expect major adjustments when people are admitted to long-term care.	Interventions can be planned to reduce resident stress and anxiety.
Address each basic human need.	All aspects of the resident's human needs will be recognized and met through appropriate nursing care planning.
Identify communication limitations and report.	Interventions can be developed to improve the free flow of interactions.

ACTIVITIES

Vocabulary Exercise. Complete the crossword puzzle by using the definitions presented.

Down

1. Disorder of the brain that involves thinking, memory, and judgment
2. Recalling past events
3. Outcomes

Across

4. Living actively
5. Name given to people in long-term care
6. Relating to teeth
7. Gas
8. Excessive urination at night

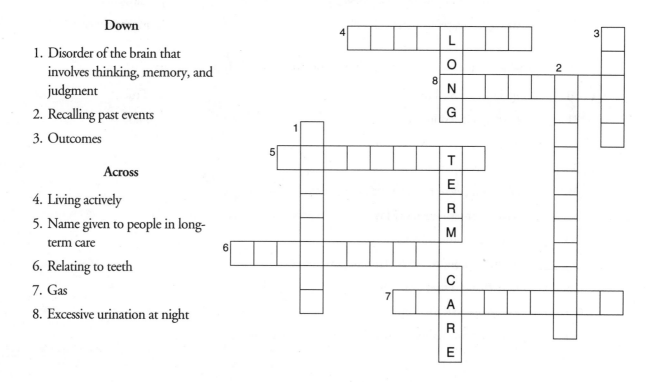

Definitions. Define the following words.

9. Medicaid _____

10. pigmentation _____

11. debilitating _____

12. assisted living _____

13. sundowning _____

14. superimpose _____

15. diverticulitis _____

16. chronological _____

17. dementia _____

18. long-term care _____

Matching. Match the words on the right with the statements on the left.

19. ____   capacity for endurance   a. prosthesis

20. ____   excessive gas in stomach or intestines   b. delegate

21. ____   assign a task to another   c. sensorium

22. ____   weakening   d. vitality

23. ____   to treat as if of less value   e. atrophy

24. ____   an artificial substitute for a missing body part   f. diverticula

25. ____   language impairment   g. debilitating

26. ____   wasting away of muscles   h. aphasia

27. ____   involuntary voiding or defecating   i. depreciate

28. ____   consciousness or mental awareness   j. flatulence

29. ____   weakened places in intestinal wall   k. incontinence

Determine which of the following are true statements about all elderly people. They:

30. ____   no longer contribute to society   a. True

31. ____   have no interest in sex   b. False

32. ____   are living in poverty

33. ____   have sensory losses

34. ____   are incompetent to make decisions

35. ____   have short-term memory loss

36. ____   undergo postural changes

37. ____   are more prone to certain chronic conditions

38. ____   have changed sleep patterns

39. ____   are unable to learn

40. ____   have the same rights as any citizen of the United States

Match resident with the proper period of adult life.

41. ___	Ethel Jamison, 72 is recovering from a brain attack.	a. early adulthood
42. ___	Julie Benson, 26, has quadriplegia following a swimming accident.	b. middle adulthood
43. ___	James McCracken, 38, who has hemiplegia is in rehabilitation after being in a skiing accident.	c. late adulthood
44. ___	Veronica Valdez, 68, has aphasia.	d. old age

41. ___ Ethel Jamison, 72 is recovering
from a brain attack.

a. early adulthood
b. middle adulthood

42. ___ Julie Benson, 26, has quadriplegia
following a swimming accident.

c. late adulthood

43. ___ James McCracken, 38, who has hemiplegia
is in rehabilitation after being in a skiing accident.

d. old age

44. ___ Veronica Valdez, 68, has aphasia.

45. ___ Brenda Thompson, 47, has paraplegia following an
automobile crash.

46. ___ Charlie Peters, 78, has Alzheimer's disease.

47. ___ Vickie Langley, 52, is recovering from brain lacerations
sustained in a fall.

48. ___ Edith Daley, 92, is disoriented due to advancing arteriosclerosis.

49. ___ Carole Brooks, 56, is undergoing bladder retraining.

50. ___ Robert Baker, 22, is in rehabilitation following a spinal cord injury.

51. ___ Harvey Penlac, 86, has diverticulosis.

Match the problem with the system affected.

52. ___ blood vessels less elastic

a. integumentary

53. ___ constipation

b. sensory

54. ___ stress incontinence

c. musculoskeletal

55. ___ less flexibility

d. urinary

56. ___ hearing diminishes

e. digestive

57. ___ primary taste sensation decreases

f. cardiovascular

58. ___ flatulence

59. ___ slower movements

60. ___ depth perception diminished

61. ___ hair loses color

Completion. Complete the following statements in the spaces provided.

62. To be successful as a long-term care nursing assistant, you must have a sense of _____ and be
able to _____ effectively.

63. Every resident must be treated with _____ .

64. Most of the residents in long-term care are _____ and have _____ health problems.

65. The long-term care nursing assistant must be satisfied with _____ progress and
_____ gains.

66. Each person moves from infancy to old age at an _____ rate.

67. Some researchers believe each person has an inborn biological _____ .

68. In the aged, response to sensory stimuli is _____ and less _____ .

69. Elderly people may not be _____ of their need for fluid.

70. Recreation and exercise should be handled at _____ times to prevent fatigue in the elderly.

71. The resident's mouth must be inspected _____ dentures are cleaned and replaced.

72. When walking and active ambulation are not feasible, range-of-motion exercises should be carried out for _____ .

73. OBRA requires all nursing assistants working in long-term care to complete a course of at least _____ clock hours.

74. Competency tests may be taken _____ times.

75. Nursing assistants must take part in ongoing _____ education.

76. Nursing assistants who are not employed for _____ months must repeat the course and competency test.

77. Manipulative behaviors are attempts to overcome feelings of _____ .

78. Frustrations at physical _____ and loss of _____ control are common among elderly.

79. Elderly people may develop an apathy about food that becomes _____ .

80. Lotions should be applied _____ to dry skin.

81. Warm baths are best given at _____ .

Brief Answers.   Answer the following questions.

82. What are three services offered by extended care facilities?

a. _____

b. _____

c. _____

83. What characteristics of the adult resident must the nursing assistant keep in mind to ensure an effective relationship?

_____

_____

_____

_____

_____

84. What are five changes frequently seen in the elderly integumentary system?

a. _____

b. _____

c. _____

d. _____

e. _____

85. What are the four basic emotion needs of the elderly?

a. _____

b. _____

c. _____

d. _____

86. The most healthy emotional responses to the process of aging are:

_____

_____

_____

_____

_____

87. What are eight ways to prevent falls when the patient has vision impairments.

a. _____   e. _____

b. _____   f. _____

c. _____   g. _____

d. _____   h. _____

88. What are five actions the nursing assistant can take to handle the problem of pillaging and hoarding?

a. _____

b. _____

c. _____

d. _____

e. _____

89. What are five reasons elderly people are prone to infections?

a. _____

b. _____

c. _____

d. _____

e. _____

90. Which resident behaviors demonstrate feelings of frustration?

a. _____

b. _____

c. _____

d. _____

e. _____

f. _____

g. _____

h. _____

i. _____

91. What are five ways the nursing assistant can help prevent infections in nursing home residents?

a. _____

b. _____

c. _____

d. _____

e. _____

92. Explain each of the activities that are associated with residents suffering from dementia.

    a. Short-term memory loss _____

    b. Complete disorientation _____

    c. Wandering _____

    d. Sundowning _____

    e. Perseveration phenomena _____

93. What is meant by a "catastrophic reaction" relating to a person with dementia?

    _____

    _____

True/False. Mark the following true or false by circling T or F.

94. T   F   Reminiscing is an inappropriate activity for elderly people.

95. T   F   Reminiscing helps people adapt to old age by allowing them to work through personal losses.

96. T   F   Reminiscing is a natural activity for people of all ages.

97. T   F   Reminiscing should be ignored because such remembrances have little relationship to today.

98. T   F   Clocks with large numbers should be placed around the facility.

99. T   F   Care for disoriented patients includes asking the residents frequently to identify the date or the caregiver.

100. T   F   Treat adult residents as children when they act confused.

101. T   F   Call residents by cute or pet names so they will feel at home.

102. T   F   Avoid confronting residents with information they may have difficulty handling.

Multiple Choice. Select the one best answer for each question.

103. Skilled nursing care facilities

    a. are known as intermediate care homes.

    b. are bed and board facilities.

    c. provide nursing care of a less acute nature.

    d. employ only registered nurses.

104. Most residents in extended care facilities

    a. are very young.

    b. have temporary acute conditions.

    c. require very little health care and supervision.

    d. have chronic, progressive conditions.

105. Characteristics of the nursing assistant that are specially important while caring for older residents include

    a. patience   c.   a sense of humor

    b. kindness   d.   all of these.

106. Characteristics of the elderly include the fact that

    a. vitality is increased.   c.   appetite is increased.

    b. night sleep is decreased.   d.   mobility and agility are increased.

107. Nocturia refers to

    a. wandering at night.   c. frequent napping.

    b. frequency of urination at night.   d. increased appetite.

108. Which of the following applies to the bath of the elderly?

    a. Full daily baths are essential

    b. Use large amounts of soap to rid the skin of dead cells

    c. Frequent bathing is essential

    d. Use deodorants liberally

109. Which of the following is true of nail care?

    a. Toenails should be cut straight across

    b. A stiff brush should be used to clean nails

    c. Fingernails should be cut straight across

    d. Thick, dry toenails can safely be filed

110. Fecal impaction is best treated by

    a. high-bulk foods.   c. oil retention enemas.

    b. decreasing exercise.   d. manual extraction.

111. Factors that help prevent accidents in long-term care facilities include:

    a. use of bright, shiny mirrors.   c. increasing the noise levels.

    b. tubs or showers with chairs.   d. using colors in the blue-green family.

112. Factors that contribute to falls by residents include the fact that older people:

    a. may have changes in vision and hearing.

    b. use medications that affect balance.

    c. do not use assistive devices properly.

    d. all of these.

Clinical Situations. Briefly describe how a nursing assistant should react to the following situations.

113. Mrs. Li, 92, is withdrawn much of the time but occasionally is complaining, hostile, and demanding. Her family seldom visits and her behavior is the same toward them.

114. Your patient reported drinking a lot of water, but the water carafe was still almost full.

115. You are about to ambulate a resident who uses a cane and you find that the rubber tip is partially broken.

Hidden Picture. Identify the problems that need attention in the picture (there are thirteen)

116. a. _____

    c. _____

    d. _____

    e. _____

    f. _____

    g. _____

    h. _____

    i. _____

    j. _____

    k. _____

    l. _____

    m. _____

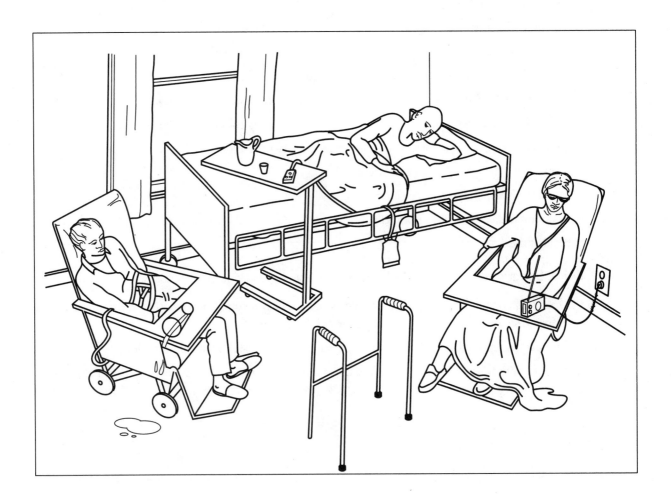

RELATING TO THE NURSING PROCESS

Write the step of the nursing process that is related to the nursing assistant action.

Nursing Assistant Action	Nursing Process Step
117. The nursing assistant reassures the people in his or her care that they will not be abandoned.	_____
118. The nursing assistant treats each resident with respect.	_____
119. The nursing assistant reports that the resident has complained of feeling constipated.	_____
120. The nursing assistant encourages the resident to feed himself but is ready to assist if needed.	_____
121. The nursing assistant encourages the resident to drink fluids frequently.	_____
122. The nursing assistant checks the cane for adequate tip tread before handing it to the resident.	_____
123. The nursing assistant uses gestures to help communicate meaning when the resident is hearing-impaired.	_____

DEVELOPING GREATER INSIGHT

124. Discuss with classmates the differences between reality orientation and validation therapy, including how each is appropriately used and the possible benefits to the resident.

125. Explain ways to protect the resident who wanders.

UNIT 32   The Organization of Home Care: Trends in Health Care

OBJECTIVES

As a result of this unit, you will be able to:

- Spell and define terms.

- Briefly describe the history of home care.

- Describe the benefits of working in home care.

- Identify members of the home health team.

- List guidelines for avoiding liability while working as a home health aide.

- Describe the types of information a home health aide must be able to document.

- Identify several time management techniques.

- List ways in which the home health aid can work successfully with families.

UNIT SUMMARY

There is an increasing trend to provide home health care to the housebound, recuperating, and chronically ill client. The nursing assistant who provides this care may also carry out some housekeeping activities.

In some situations, the duties are specifically separated into household and personal tasks performed by a homemaker assistant and the nursing care activities performed by the home health care nursing assistant.

Home health care consists of:

- Maintaining a safe, comfortable environment for the client.

- Managing infection control.

- Carrying out proper nursing techniques under the supervision of the nurse care coordinator.

The home health assistant occupies the position of:

- Member of the home health care team.

- Guest in the client's home.

- Provider of direct health care and household assistance.

NURSING ASSISTANT ALERT

Action	Benefit
Document according to agency policy.	Provides accurate information regarding caregiver, client progress, and financial costs.
Know agency nursing assistant job description and carry out those responsibilities only.	Avoids liability and assures cost reimbursement.
Know and support client's rights.	Assures that client will be treated with respect and dignity.

ACTIVITIES

Vocabulary Exercise. Write the definition for each of the following.

1. Client care records _____

2. Intermediate care _____

3. Time travel records _____

Completion. Complete the following statements in the spaces provided. Select the correct term from the list provided.

accuracy	assistance	calculations	complete
developed	home health care team	hospital	independence
insurance group	number	nurse	one
part-time	records	skilled care facility	taught

4. An advantage to working as a nursing assistant in the home is that there are opportunities for _____ employment.

5. In home care there is the opportunity to give _____ care to _____ client at a time.

6. The home health care aide has an opportunity to work with greater _____.

7. The care of the client is planned by the _____.

8. The services of the home nursing assistant may be a referral from a/an _____.

9. It is important to keep accurate time and cost _____ of the care you give.

10. Most persons using home care have been discharged from a/an _____ or _____.

11. Clients may be in need of _____ with activities of daily living.

12. A nursing assistant may be assigned to care for a client for a _____ of hours daily.

13. The care plan is _____ with the client by the _____.

14. Liability can be avoided if the nursing assistant carries out actions as he or she was _____.

15. Keeping time/travel records requires _____ and _____.

Brief Answers. Briefly answer the following questions in the spaces provided.

16. Name three different types of home care providers.

    a. _____

    b. _____

    c. _____

17. List four advantages to working for a home health agency.

    a. _____

    b. _____

    c. _____

    d. _____

18. What are five time and cost values to record?

    a. _____

    b. _____

    c. _____

    d. _____

    e. _____

19. What are included in the client care records?

    a. _____

    b. _____

    c. _____

20. What are five ways to avoid liability when providing home care?

    a. _____

    b. _____

    c. _____

    d. _____

    e. _____

21. What are four sources for reimbursement of costs for home care?

    a. _____

    b. _____

    c. _____

    d. _____

22. What are four types of activities that should be included in the client care record?

    a. _____

    b. _____

    c. _____

    d. _____

23. What are five steps you can take to help manage time at the client's home?

    a. _____

b. _____

c. _____

d. _____

e. _____

Matching. Match the activity or responsibility with the proper home health team member.

Activity/Responsibility

24. ___ May or may not be supportive of client.

25. ___ Writes orders and acts as a consultant and guide.

26. ___ Provides direct client care.

27. ___ Person in need of care.

28. ___ May act as alternate caregivers.

29. ___ Provides for client's safety and comfort.

30. ___ Makes observations about care that was given.

31. ___ Teaches and supervises nursing assistants.

32. ___ Requires skilled services.

33. ___ Plans care.

34. ___ May require assistance with ADLs.

35. ___ Completes periodic client assessments.

36. ___ Documents observations and care that was given.

37. ___ May live in the client's home.

Health Care Team

a. client

b. family

c. nursing assistant

d. supervising nurse

e. physician

Computations.

38. Compute the time spent in each case.

Arrival Time		Departure Time		Time Spent
a. 8:15 AM	_____	8:50 AM	_____	_____
b. 10:05 AM	_____	11:15 AM	_____	_____
c. 11:20 AM	_____	1:05 PM	_____	_____
d. 2:10 PM	_____	3:15 PM	_____	_____
e. 3:45 PM	_____	4:30 PM	_____	_____

Clinical Situations. Briefly describe what the nursing assistant could do to meet the following needs in the home setting.

39. Mary Johnson, who is 78 years of age, has diabetes mellitus. She requires a bed bath, change of linens, and a blood glucose level check. Your arrival time is 8:20 AM and you leave the client's home at 9:05. Your odometer read 42,738 miles when you left the agency and 42,743 miles when you arrived at the client's home. Compute the time spent with the client and the mileage from the agency to the client's home.

_____

_____

40. Mr. Alleandra is 58 and has a diagnosis of terminal cancer of the bone. Your assignment is to spend an entire evening shift with him. In addition to feeding the client and meeting his comfort needs, the family wishes Mr. Alleandra to have company. He likes to play cards and dominos and to watch TV. Describe your actions.

_____

_____

41. Mrs. Parks has congestive heart failure and tires so easily that she has difficulty carrying out her daily living activities. You are assigned to assist her for an entire shift. The family wants you to wash the floor and windows, vacuum, and do the laundry. These actions are not part of the nursing assistant's job description.

_____

_____

RELATING TO THE NURSING PROCESS

Write the step of the nursing process that is related to the nursing assistant action.

Nursing Assistant Action	Nursing Process Step
42. The nursing assistant performs only skills she has been taught when providing home care.	_____
43. The nursing assistant and the supervisor discuss the exact care to be given to the homebound client.	_____
44. The nursing assistant keeps careful records of the length of time spent on specific activities when in the client's home.	_____

DEVELOPING GREATER INSIGHT

45. You are assigned to work the night shift in Mrs. Lawrence's home. The client sleeps most of the night but must be awakened to take her medication at 12 midnight and 4 AM. Think what activities you might engage in while the client sleeps.

46. Discuss with classmates the reasons why clients might prefer to have home care rather than remain in a long-term care facility.

47. Invite a nursing assistant who works in home care to share his or her experiences with you.

UNIT 33   The Nursing Assistant in Home Care

OBJECTIVES

As a result of this unit, you will be able to:
- Spell and define terms.
- Describe the characteristics that are especially important tot he nursing assistant providing home care.
- Describe the duties of the nursing assistant who works in the home setting.
- Describe the duties of the homemaker assistant.
- Carry out home care activities needed to maintain a safe and clean environment.

UNIT SUMMARY

There is an increasing trend to provide home health care to housebound, recuperating, and chronically ill clients. The nursing assistant who provides this care may also carry out housekeeping activities.

Home health care consists of:
- Maintaining a safe, comfortable environment for the client.
- Managing infection control.
- Carrying out proper nursing techniques under the supervision of the nurse care coordinator.

The home health assistant occupies the position of a:
- Member of the home health care team.
- Guest in the client's home.
- Provider of direct health care and household assistance.

NURSING ASSISTANT ALERT

Action	Benefit
Adapt procedures to the home setting following accepted technique and safety standards.	Ensures that the same standard of care will be given in all health care settings.
Carry out housekeeping duties diligently.	Secures a clean and safe environment for the client.
Be alert to unsafe conditions in the home.	Avoids injury to client and caregiver.
Adapt procedures to equipment found in the home whenever possible.	Contributes to cost containment.

ACTIVITIES

Vocabulary Exercise. Put a circle around word defined.

1. another name for a home health care aide.

2. another name for the homemaker assistant

3. another name for the home health assistant

4. another name for the homemaker aide

```
N D R E Y N T C L M D H Y K V X B W D N G P
U P A J Z K D W S B X T E R G S D P A O S W
K O T G L M U O P K C D I U L T J N H Y T F
W N H O S N I R P Y I V J W P L F Q C L B T
B R E N Y T X B X A R L E B Z N J M D S U G
J E Q L A K F E R N S D F T I Q O K T J W M
I Z H O M E H E A L T H A S S I S T A N T Z
C R X J S L K Q K U T C H F X B Y U D R O N
I L P E D I A H T L A E H E M O(H)M O B A K
O Y C D M R E X N U P N G D P C S N G W I Q
N F T E H M D I V L K A M I J Y A A R E C L
U D M Q N S L A Y M R Z L C J H N S K S O K
H O M E M A K E R A S S I S T A N T E F N Z
H T I B G T P J S G W D U M W E S L V L J M
```

Completion. Complete the following statements in the spaces provided.

5. The nursing assistant contributes to the planning step of the nursing process by actively participating in _____.

6. The client should, if able, make decisions about food _____.

7. The client's bathroom should be cleaned _____.

8. Before _____ the client's appliances, seek _____ from a family member.

9. Be sure to _____ the _____ off before hanging laundered clothes outside.

10. Before storing clothes that have been laundered, check for needed _____.

11. Drip-dry fabrics should be washed _____ so they can be hung and folded.

12. The primary role of the home health assistant is to _____.

13. The major responsibility of the homemaker assistant is to provide _____.

14. The nursing assistant providing health care may be asked in some cases to carry out _____ chores.

15. Because home health assistants handle money, they must be _____ people.

16. The home health care assistant activities are planned around the _____.

17. To save costs, _____ enema equipment may substituted for disposable enema equipment.

18. Statements of the client that reflect neglect or abuse should be _____.

19. Chemicals such as household cleaning supplies and insecticides should be kept locked up when the client is

_____ .

20. Dust, dirty dishes, and improperly caring for foods contribute to the spread of _____.

Brief Answers. Briefly answer the following questions in the spaces provided.

21. What are three areas to report that support the assessment process?

a. _____

b. _____

c. _____

22. What are two ways to support the implementation portion of the nursing process?

   a. _____

   b. _____

23. What are two ways to promote the evaluation part of the nursing process?

   a. _____

   b. _____

24. What are nine characteristics of the home nursing assistant?

   a. _____

   b. _____

   c. _____

   d. _____

   e. _____

   f. _____

   g. _____

   h. _____

   i. _____

25. What are three household duties the nursing assistant frequently performs?

   a. _____

   b. _____

   c. _____

26. What are three household cleaning duties not included in the nursing assistant's responsibilities?

   a. _____

   b. _____

   c. _____

27. What are four numbers to be kept close to the phone during home care?

   a. _____

   b. _____

   c. _____

   d. _____

28. What guidelines should be kept in mind when making food purchases for the client?

   a. _____

   b. _____

   c. _____

   d. _____

   e. _____

   f. _____

29. What action should be nursing assistant take when cleaning laundry soiled by blood?

   _____

30. How can wastepaper baskets be kept cleaner and less a source of infection?

    a. _____

    b. _____

    c. _____

31. How should the client's dishes be washed by hand?

    a. _____

    b. _____

    c. _____

    d. _____

    e. _____

True/False. Mark the following true or false by circling T or F.

32. T   F   Household duties may be part of the home nursing assistant's responsibilities.

33. T   F   Caring for food properly is part of your responsibility.

34. T   F   It is all right to leave dirty dishes in the sink after the client eats.

35. T   F   Cleaning the client's bathroom and kitchen are part of the nursing assistant's responsibilities.

36. T   F   Fresh fruits that are to be used right away should be stored in the refrigerator.

37. T   F   Dried and canned foods should be stored in the refrigerator.

38. T   F   It is proper to leave dairy products unrefrigerated until use.

39. T   F   Frozen foods may be safely thawed in the kitchen sink until use.

40. T   F   Dirty dishes left to accumulate will contribute to infection.

41. T   F   Loose scatter rugs are safe to use in the home if the client knows where they are placed.

42. T   F   Electrical outlets which have multiple cords plugged in could cause fires.

Clinical Situations. Briefly describe what the nursing assistant could do to meet the following needs in the home setting.

43. The bed is not flexible and the client needs to be in a semi-Fowler's position.

    _____

44. The client has sprained an ankle and there is no ice bag to apply cold.

    _____

    _____

45. The client needs to remain in bed and likes to do puzzles to pass the time.

    _____

46. The client is very heavy and there is no trapeze to help with lifting and moving.

    _____

47. You must give a bed bath and there is no bath blanket.

    _____

48. The client must remain in bed, so all care must be given on a regular-height twin bed.

    _____

49. The client is a child who, though in traction, has many toys, crayons, and books scattered over the bed.

_____

50. You need a place to put soiled laundry as you give care.

_____

51. The client needs occasional enemas, and disposable enema equipment is too expensive.

_____

52. The client has an upper respiratory infection, and you must safely dispose of soiled tissues.

_____

_____

53. You are visiting Mrs. Morrison regularly as part of your assignment. This morning you notice a bruise on her arm and she tells you that she and her daughter, who lives with her, quarreled last evening. What action should you take.

_____

_____

54. Mary Schroeder is 91 years of age and is very frail. She has been diagnosed with emphysema, CHF, and diabetes. She is cared for by her sister, who is 93 years of age. You are assigned to provide personal hygiene care three mornings each week. Ms. Schroeder is in a regular bed that is low to the floor and cannot have its position changed. The client is incontinent. You must adapt her low-income environment to provide proper care.

_____

_____

_____

RELATING TO THE NURSING PROCESS

Write the step of the nursing process that is related to the nursing assistant action.

Nursing Assistant Action	Nursing Process Step
55. The nursing assistant reports to her supervisor improvement in the homebound client's appetite.	_____
56. The nursing assistant reports that the client receiving home care is now able to function independently.	_____
57. The nursing assistant informs the supervisor that stress between client and daughter about the client's planned activities is interfering with the client's performance.	_____

DEVELOPING GREATER INSIGHT

58. Think back to a time when you were under extreme stress. Did you strike out physically or verbally and then were sorry afterward?

59. Make out a shopping list for meals for one day for two people who are on unrestricted diets but limited income. Look through newspapers for coupons and sales that could save money.

60. Look carefully around your own home and try to identify safety factors that could be changed if health care were needed.

UNIT 34   Subacute Care

OBJECTIVES

As a result of this unit, you will be able to:
- Spell and define terms.
- Describe the purpose of subacute care.
- List the differences between acute care, subacute care, and long-term care.
- Describe the responsibilities of the nursing assistant when caring for patients receiving the special treatments in subacute care.
- Demonstrate the following procedure:

    Procedure 91 Changing a Gown on a Patient with a Peripheral Intravenous Line in Place

UNIT SUMMARY

Nursing assistants working in subacute care units must have an advanced education and experience caring for the types of patients found in these units. They must be able to support complex therapies while providing basic nursing care.

Nursing assistants must be prepared to give assistance in the care of patients receiving special therapy such as:
- Chemotherapy.
- Rehabilitation.
- Central venous insertion.
- Intravenous therapy.
- Total parenteral nutrition.
- Patient-controlled analgesia (PAC).
- Epidural catheter approach to pain management.
- Transcutaneous electrical nerve stimulation (TENS).
- Tracheostomy.
- Radiation.
- Hemodialysis.

Nursing assistants must know:
- The purpose of the therapy.
- Important observations to report.
- Special nursing care techniques.

NURSING ASSISTANT ALERT

Action	Benefit
Participate in in-service education classes.	Develops skills needed to meet specific patient needs.
Seek information in textbooks about the specific conditions and care of the types of patients in the unit.	Increases understanding of the reasons for and ways special techniques are carried out.
Participate in interdisciplinary team conferences.	Increase understanding of specific patients and their care. Assures that individual patient will receive optimum care.

ACTIVITIES

Vocabulary Exercise. Match the terms on the right with the definitions on the left.

1. ___	Care and treatment of persons with cancer	a. alopecia
2. ___	Drugs given to relieve severe pain	b. anorexia
3. ___	Additional bag of fluid added to the main IV line	c. chemotherapy
4. ___	Artificial opening in trachea	d. fistula
5. ___	Subacute care	e. graft
6. ___	Loss of hair	f. narcotic
7. ___	Created when a vein is attached to an artery in an arm or leg	g. oncology
8. ___	Use of drugs to kill cancer cells in the body	h. piggyback
9. ___	Loss of appetite	i. tracheostomy
10. ___	Synthetic material inserted to form a connection between an artery and a vein	j. transitional care

Completion. Complete the following statements in the spaces provided. Select the proper terms from the list provided.

approaches	areas	consistency	emotional
goals	hyperalimentation	participate	peripheral
skilled nursing	transitional	3 to 4 weeks	

11. Some acute care is sometimes referred to as _____ care.

12. Subacute care units are usually located in _____ facilities.

13. Most patients remain in a subacute unit for _____.

14. Most subacute care units provide specialized care in one or two _____.

15. Nursing assistants _____ in special in-service education to meet the needs of subacute care patients.

16. Nursing assistants provide for the _____ well-being of the patients.

17. To give proper care, the nursing assistant must know that _____ have been established.

18. The key to successful rehabilitation is _____.

19. IV therapy refers to fluids and medications given directly into a _____ vein.

20. TPN is also called _____.

Brief Answers. Briefly answer each question in the spaces provided.

21. What is the purpose of subacute care?

_____

_____

22. Where do patients continue their care after discharge from a subacute care unit?

a. _____

b. _____

c. _____

23. What are five expectations of a nursing assistant working on a subacute care unit?

a. _____

b. _____

c. _____

d. _____

e. _____

24. What are three types of patient who may require intensive rehabilitation?

a. _____

b. _____

c. _____

25. What are two reasons IV therapy is administered with a central venous catheter?

a. _____

b. _____

26. What do the letters PICC stand for?

_____

27. What are four actions the nursing assistant must *not* take when caring for a patient with an IV?

a. _____

b. _____

c. _____

d. _____

28. What are five important observations you should make when caring for a patient who is on dialysis?

a. _____

b. _____

c. _____

d. _____

e. _____

29. What are four important observations to report about a patient receiving epidural catheter pain relief?

   a. _____

   b. _____

   c. _____

   d. _____

30. What are four observations that should be reported related to the patient with a tracheostomy?

   a. _____

   b. _____

   c. _____

   d. _____

Completion. Complete the following related to care of the patient receiving an IV..

31. Know the _____ rate.

32. Notify the nurse if the drip chamber is _____ .

33. Avoid twisting or pulling _____ .

34. Make sure patient does not _____ on the tubing.

35. Observe needle insertion for signs of _____ .

36. Make sure all _____ in tubing are secure.

37. Note signs of moisture that might indicate _____ .

38. Report signs of _____ , _____ , chest or back pain.

True/False. Mark the following true or false by circling T or F.

39. T F Some patients may feel very uncertain when in a subacute care unit.

40. T F Pulse oximetry is used to monitor the pulse rate.

41. T F The pulse oximeter is placed over the patient's heart.

42. T F Never allow the bag of IV fluid to be lower than the patient's arm.

43. T F The dosage for PAC is controlled by equipment that is preset by the nurse.

44. T F An epidural catheter is implanted under the skin near the elbow to administer a local anesthetic.

45. T F Dialysis is the process of cleansing liquid wastes artificially from the body.

46. T F Radiation therapy uses high-energy radiation.

47. T F TENS is a nondrug method of pain relief.

48. T F Heat or cold treatments can be applied directly over an area being radiated.

49. T F Chemotherapy is always administered through the IV route.

50. T F Patients with tracheostomies should be cautioned about using shaving cream around the stoma.

Clinical Situations. Briefly describe how a nursing assistant should react to the following situations.

51. Mr. Riggs is on your unit with renal failure due to mercury poisoning. He has a graft that is used for his hemodialysis treatments. Describe the special care you will give him.

   a. _____

   b. _____

c. _____

d. _____

e. _____

52. Mrs. Ford is being treated with radiation for metastatic pancreatic cancer. She has markings on her skin for treatment purposes. What care should be taken of these marks?

53. Mrs. Johns is receiving chemotherapy for cancer of the lungs. She receives her drugs orally. She is complaining of nausea and is vomiting.

RELATING TO THE NURSING PROCESS

Write the step of the nursing process that is related to the nursing assistant action.

Nursing Assistant Action	**Nursing Process Step**
54. The nursing assistant reports that her patient, who is receiving chemotherapy by IV has a reddened area at the site of the needle insertion.	_____
55. The nursing assistant reports that the patient, who has an epidural catheter for pain relief, is complaining of numbness in her right leg.	_____
56. The nursing assistant carefully monitors the patient's vital signs following peritoneal dialysis.	_____

DEVELOPING GREATER INSIGHT

57. Invite a nursing assistant who works in subacute care to discuss his or her experiences with you.

58. Visit a subacute care unit. If possible:

   a. Observe a working assistant.

   b. Identify the types of patients on the unit.

59. Return to the classroom and discuss your experiences with your classmates and instructor.

UNIT 35   Integumentary System

OBJECTIVES

As a result of this unit, you will be able to:

- Spell and define terms.

- Review the location and function of the skin.

- Describe some common skin lesions.

- List three diagnostic tests associated with skin conditions.

- Describe the nursing assistant actions relating to the nursing care of patients with specific skin conditions.

- Identify persons at risk for the formation of pressure ulcers.

- Describe measures to prevent pressure ulcers.

- Describe the stages of pressure ulcer formation and identify appropriate nursing assistant actions.

- List nursing assistant actions in caring for patients with burns.

UNIT SUMMARY

- The condition of the skin indicates the general health of the body. The presence of conditions are revealed through skin:

  Color.
  Texture.
  Lesions or eruptions.

- Pressure ulcers result from pressure on one area of the body that interferes with circulation. Pressure ulcers:

  Are more easily prevented than cured.
  May occur in any patient.
  Occur in stages that are recognizable and treatable.

- Burns:

  Are classified according to the depth of tissue damage.
  Require special care, often in burn centers.

- Burn therapy involves:

  Analgesics for pain.
  Infection control.
  Replacement of lost fluids and electrolytes.
  Possible skin grafting to repair injured tissue.
  Position changes and support to prevent contractures an deformities.

NURSING ASSISTANT ALERT

Action	Benefit
Observe and carefully describe skin lesions.	Establishes proper data for more accurate evaluation.
Identify those patients at risk for pressure ulcers.	Allows timely nursing interventions
Carry out pressure ulcer care as prescribed.	Limits more extensive involvement. Promotes repair.

ACTIVITIES

Vocabulary Exercise. Define the following words.

1. cyanotic _____

2. crust _____

3. debride _____

4. obese _____

5. rubra _____

6. contraindicated _____

7. allergy _____

8. lesions _____

9. pallor _____

10. necrosis _____

Anatomy Review. Name the areas indicated by writing their proper names in the spaces provided.

11. _____

12. _____

13. _____

14. _____

15. _____

16. _____

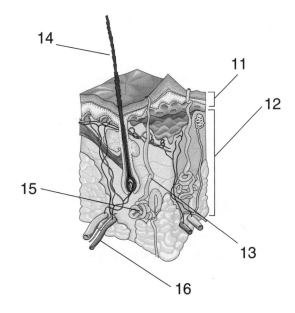

Completion. Complete the following statements in the spaces provided.

17. Another name for allergies is _____ reactions.

18. The most severe allergic reaction is called _____ shock.

19. Soap and water are often _____ when there are multiple skin lesions.

20. Patients with skin lesions must be handled _____ without _____ the skin.

21. Pressure ulcers are more easily _____ than _____ .

22. Pressure ulcers are common in obese patients under the _____ , in the abdominal folds, and between the folds of the _____ .

23. Reddened skin is a sign of the _____ stage of tissue breakdown.

24. If the epidermis is broken, it should be kept _____

25. Indication of infection in a pressure ulcer might include _____ and a foul _____ .

26. Early necrosis over a pressure point may be indicated by redness or _____ discoloration.

27. In stage II breakdown, it is imperative that the _____ be relieved or more serious damage will occur.

28. Daily _____ baths help keep open pressure ulcers clean.

29. In severe cases of Stage III pressure ulcers, it may be necessary to perform _____ to close the lesion.

30. Skin lesions may be caused by _____ .

31. Crusts should not be removed from skin lesions without _____ .

32. Shearing occurs when skin moves in one direction while structures underneath _____ .

33. Patients with Stage V pressure ulcers experience _____ and _____ and are at great risk for infection.

34. Elevating the head of the bed no higher than _____ helps prevent shearing.

35. A patient who is sitting in a geri-chair should be encouraged to raise himself or herself every _____ _____ .

Brief Answers. Briefly answer the following questions.

36. What clinical problem might you suspect because of these changes in skin?

    a. hot, dry flushed _____

    b. darkish blue, cyanotic_____

    c. very dry _____

37. How could you best document the following skin lesions?

    a. flat discolored as in measles_____

    b. skin appears scratched or scraped away _____

    c. raised spot filled with serous fluid _____

    d. areas of dried body secretions _____

38. Which four types of patients are prone to tissue breakdown?

    a. _____

    b. _____

    c. _____

    d. _____

39. What are twelve ways to avoid the development of pressure ulcers?

    a. _____

    b. _____

    c. _____

    d. _____

    e. _____

    f. _____

    g. _____

    h. _____

    i. _____

    j. _____

    k. _____

    l. _____

40. What are the four goals of burn treatment?

    a. _____

    b. _____

    c. _____

    d. _____

41. What special care will the nursing assistant emphasize when assisting in the care of a burn patient?

    a. _____

    b. _____

    c. _____

    d. _____

    e. _____

    f. _____

42. What four actions can the nursing assistant take to increase circulation to tissues?

a. _____

b. _____

c. _____

d. _____

43. Why is it important to avoid creating skin tears?

a. _____

b. _____

c. _____

44. Mr. French is in fair physical condition. He is rather lethargic and is ambulatory with assistance. He has limited movement of his left arm and leg, is continent and eats poorly. He has an open lesion over his left hip. What is risk of pressure sore development?

_____

45. Complete the turning wheel to demonstrate your understanding of the principle of relieving pressure.

46. List the areas most subject to breakdown when the patient is in the position shown.

a. _____

b. _____

c. _____

d. _____

e. _____

Clinical Situations. Briefly describe how a nursing assistant should react to the following situations.

47. You burned your finger.

_____

48. You are assigned to give a bed bath and find the patient has skin lesions.

_____

_____

RELATING TO THE NURSING PROCESS

Write the step of the nursing process that is related to the nursing assistant action.

Nursing Assistant Action	Nursing Process Step
49. The nursing assistant charts the presence of excoriations on the patient's chest.	_____
50. The nursing assistant gently massages outside a reddened area, following the nurse's orders.	_____
51. The nursing assistant reports a pustule noted on the patient's thigh.	_____
52. The nursing assistant makes sure the patient's position is changed at least every two hours.	_____
53. The nursing assistant uses a turning sheet to move dependent patients in bed.	_____
54. The nursing assistant reports an area of irritation around the entrance of the nasogastric tube into the nose.	_____

DEVELOPING GREATER INSIGHT

55. What do the following patients have in common: a patient with a nasogastric tube, a patient with an indwelling catheter, and a patient who is able to move independently?

56. Discuss with classmates reasons why changes in the aging integumentary system make the elderly more prone to develop pressure ulcers.

UNIT 36   Respiratory System

OBJECTIVES

As a result of this unit, you will be able to:

- Spell and define terms.

- Review the location and function of the respiratory organs.

- Describe some common diseases of the respiratory system.

- List five diagnostic tests used to identify respiratory conditions.

- Describe nursing assistant actions related to the care of patients with respiratory conditions.

- List five safety measures for the use of oxygen therapy.

- Demonstrate the following procedure:

    Procedure 92 Refilling the Humidifier Bottle
    Procedure 93 Collecting a sputum Specimen

UNIT SUMMARY

The organs of respiration function to take in and exchange oxygen and output carbon dioxide. Diseases that affect the respiratory tract make breathing difficult. These conditions include:

- Upper respiratory infections.

- Chronic obstructive pulmonary diseases (COPD).

Special techniques that can make breathing easier include:

- Oxygen therapy.

- Incentive spirometry.

- Positioning.

- Mouth care.

Special precautions must be taken to avoid transmission of disease. These precautions include handwashing, disposing of soiled tissues and avoiding coughing and sneezing the direction of others. Observations that should be reported and documented include:

- Rate and rhythm of respiration.

- Changes in skin color.

- Character and presence of respiratory secretions.

- Cough, including character (for example, amount, color, and odor of sputum, if present).

NURSING ASSISTANT ALERT

Action	Benefit
Use standard precautions when working with patients who have respiratory tract conditions.	Prevents transmission of disease.
Note, report, and document alteration in respiratory patterns or function.	Early interventions care improve ventilation and exchange.
Be prepared to react quickly and correctly to prevent emergencies involving oxygen use.	Averts possible fire hazards and patient injury.
Follow procedures for sputum specimen collection carefully.	Avoids contamination of specimens. Protects against transmission of infectious materials.
Label and deliver sputum specimens promptly.	Prevents deterioration of specimens that might give false results.
Label specimens correctly.	Matches the proper findings with the correct patient.

ACTIVITIES

Vocabulary Exercise. Complete the puzzle by filling in the missing letters of words found in this unit. Use the definitions to help you discover these words.

1. difficult breathing

2. bringing up material from lungs

3. inspiration followed by expiration

4.

5. bluish discoloration of skin due to lack of oxygen

6. serious inflammation of the lungs

7. exchange units of the lungs

8. sensitivity reaction

9. gas needed for life

10. voice box

1. _ _ S _ _ _ _

2. _ _ P _ _ _ _ _ _ _ _

3. _ _ _ _ I _ _ _ _ _ _ _

4. R

5. _ _ _ _ O _ _ _

6. _ _ _ _ M _ _ _ _

7. _ _ _ E _ _ _

8. _ _ T _ _ _

9. _ _ _ _ E _

10. _ _ R _ _ _

Definitions. Define the following terms or abbreviations.

11. biopsy_____

12. phlegm_____

13. URI _____

14. SOB_____

15. COPD _____

16. antipyretic _____

17. arrest _____

18. croupette _____

Anatomy Review. Using a colored pencil or crayon, fill in the areas through which oxygen must flow from the outside to the exchange area. Then name the parts in their proper order.

19. a. _____

    b. _____

    c. _____

    d. _____

    e. _____

    f. _____

    g. _____

Completion. Complete the following statements in the spaces provided.

20. The patient experiencing an asthmatic attack has dyspnea and wheezing because there is increased _____ production, spasm of the _____ tree and swelling of the _____ lining the respiratory tract.

21. The person with bronchitis has _____ cough.

22. Common allergens include pollen, medications, dust, _____ and _____ .

23. Symptoms of an URI include runny nose, watery eyes, and _____ .

24. The tiny air sacs forming the lungs are called _____ .

25. In emphysema, the alveoli lose some of their _____ .

26. Changes in emphysema allow _____ to become trapped in the lungs.

27. The patient with emphysema has the most difficulty in the _____ phase of respiration.

28. It is important for the nursing assistant to know and read the _____ rate of oxygen for each patient.

29. Tent oxygen is primarily used when _____ is also needed.

30. The area around the mask during oxygen administration should be periodically _____ and

    _____ .

31. It is important to remember that a child in a croupette may suffer _____

    _____ .

Brief Answers. Briefly answer each question in the spaces provided.

32. What four practices should be taught to all patients with upper respiratory infections?

    a. _____

    b. _____

    c. _____

    d. _____

33. What are four observations regarding patients with respiratory disease that must be reported?

34. What are ten important points included in the care of patients with COPD?

    a. _____

    b. _____

    c. _____

    d. _____

    e. _____

    f. _____

    g. _____

    h. _____

    i. _____

    j. _____

35. What precautions must be taken when a patient receives oxygen from a tank?

    a. _____

    b. _____

    c. _____

    d. _____

36. The alignment of the patient in a high-Fowler's position is best supported by:

    a. _____

    b. _____

    c. _____

37. Give three characteristics of the orthopneic position.

   a. _____

   b. _____

   c. _____

38. What are three kinds of breathing exercises that may be ordered for the COPD patient?

   a. _____

   b. _____

   c. _____

39. What are two other techniques beside mucolytic medications used to loosen mucus and clear the air passageways?

   a. _____

   b. _____

Hidden Picture. Carefully study the picture below and identify the rules of oxygen safety that have been violated. Write them in the spaces provided.

40. a. _____

   b. _____

   c. _____

   d. _____

   e. _____

   f. _____

   g. _____

   h. _____

Clinical Situations. Briefly describe how a nursing assistant should react to the following situations.

41. You enter a patient's room and find the patient receiving a higher level oxygen than is ordered.

_____

42. Your patient complains of mouth dryness while receiving oxygen therapy.

_____

43. Your patient receiving oxygen therapy wants to shave with an electric razor.

_____

_____

44. You are assigned to collect a sputum specimen. Before collecting a specimen, the patient should _____ .

45. Complete the following label which is attached to a specimen container, using the following information: Mr. James Brown is a patient in room 604. His hospital number is 689473. Dr. Smith has ordered a sputum specimen to be taken today for culture.

Name_____   Room_____

Date_____   Hospital Number_____

Doctor_____

Specimen_____   Examination_____

RELATING TO THE NURSING PROCESS

Write the step of the nursing process that is related to the nursing assistant action.

Nursing Assistant Action	**Nursing Process Step**
46. The nursing assistant makes sure the strap holding a nasal cannula delivering oxygen is not too tight.	_____
47. The nursing assistant periodically removes an oxygen delivery mask and washes and dries carefully underneath it.	_____
48. The nursing assistant reports that the patient's respirations have become labored.	_____
49. The nursing assistant keeps the patient's face free of any nasal discharge when a nasal catheter is in use.	_____
50. The nursing assistant positions pillows behind the patient's back to assist his breathing.	_____
51. The nursing assistant helps position the patient as the respiratory therapist carries out chest percussion.	_____
52. The nursing assistant informs the nurse that the oxygen flowmeter is set lower than the level the nursing assistant had been given as proper during report.	_____

DEVELOPING GREATER INSIGHT

53. Try putting an oxygen mask on your face for 20 minutes. Be sure the tubing is open so you have a continuous source of air. Describe your feelings when you remove the mask.

54. In the clinical area, practice identifying the number of liters on a flowmeter under supervision.

UNIT 37   Circulatory (Cardiovascular) System

OBJECTIVES

As a result of this unit, you will be able to:
- Spell and define terms.
- Review the location and functions of the organs of the circulatory system.
- List five specific diagnostic tests for disorders of the circulatory system.
- Describe some common disorders of the circulatory system.
- Describe nursing assistant actions related to care of patients with disorders of the circulatory system.

UNIT SUMMARY

The cardiovascular system is the transportation system of the body.
- The heart and blood vessels make up a closed network. This network carries the blood and the products of and for metabolism.
- Diseases can affect the heart or blood vessels with a related effect on many parts of the body, especially the respiratory tract.
- Because heart disease is so prevalent, the nursing assistant will likely provide care for many patients with cardiovascular problems.

NURSING ASSISTANT ALERT

Action	Benefit
Do nothing to limit circulation.	Allows patient to make optimum use of cardiovascular function.
Recognize that abnormalities in any part of the cardiovascular system may affect other parts of the body as a whole.	Alerts staff to the significance of signs and symptoms that may be demonstrated in other systems.
Carefully observe, report, and document observations.	Provides a database for appropriate nursing interventions.

ACTIVITIES

Vocabulary Exercise. Unscramble the words introduced in this unit and define them.

1. N A M E A I _____

2. T O A R A _____

3. E B L S M U O _____

4. C E S H I I M A _____

5. H T M R U B O S _____

6. P R Y T O H Y E P R H _____

7. I N G N A A _____

8. D E U I S R I S _____

9. T R H M A A E O _____

10. Y R I D S S A A S C _____

Anatomy Review. Name the valves located between:

11. the right atrium and right ventricle _____

12. the left atrium and left ventricle _____

13. the right ventricle and pulmonary artery _____

14. the left ventricle and aorta _____

15. Using colored pencils or crayons, color the venous blood blue and the arterial blood red in the following figure at left.

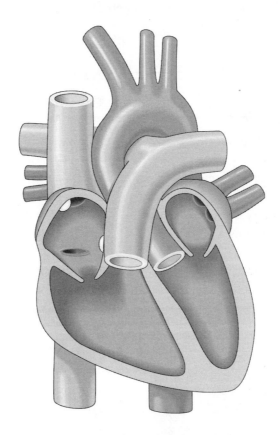

15. Name the arteries indicated in the spaces provided. Then use a red pencil or crayon to trace the pathway of blood from the heart to the left hand and left foot.

16. _____

17. _____

18. _____

19. ____heart_____

20. _____

21. _____

22. _____

23. _____

24. _____

25. _____

26. _____

Completion. Complete the following statements in the spaces provided.

27. Patients who have long-standing cardiac disease often develop diseases of the _____ system and the _____ system.

28. Blood vessels that serve the outer parts of the body are called _____ blood vessels.

29. Blood abnormalities are referred to as blood _____ .

30. Following prescribed exercises carefully can help promote _____ flow and _____ return.

31. Hypertension is another name for _____ .

32. The diet of the hypertensive usually limits the amount of _____ intake.

33. Angioplasty is a surgical procedure to _____ blood vessels.

34. Coronary bypass is a surgical procedure that _____ blocked arteries.

35. When the coronary muscles are blocked, the heart tissue becomes _____

_____ .

Brief Answers. Briefly answer the following questions.

36. Which observations would be reported about patients with circulatory disorders?

    a. _____

    b. _____

    c. _____

    d. _____

    e. _____

37. What six signs and symptoms indicate decreased circulation to an area?

    a. _____   d. _____

    b. _____   e. _____

    c. _____   f. _____

38. To what part of the body do the vessels lead that are most commonly affected by atherosclerosis and the formation of atheromas?

    a. _____

    b. _____

    c. _____

39. What seven conditions predispose a person to the development of atherosclerosis?

    a. _____

    b. _____

    c. _____

    d. _____

    e. _____

    f. _____

    g. _____

40. What four factors are stressed in the treatment for the patient with atherosclerosis?

    a. _____

    b. _____

    c. _____

    d. _____

41. What four diagnostic medical terms are used to indicate a coronary heart attack?

    a. _____

    b. _____

    c. _____

    d. _____

42. What three special observations must the nursing assistant note when caring for a patient recovering from an MI?

    a. _____

    b. _____

    c. _____

43. What four signs or symptoms might be noted and reported in the patient with CHF?

    a. _____

    b. _____

    c. _____

    d. _____

44. What seven nursing care procedures would the nursing assistant carry out for the patient with CHF?

    a. _____

    b. _____

    c. _____

    d. _____

    e. _____

    f. _____

    g. _____

True/False. Mark the following true or false by circling T or F.

45. T   F   A rocking bed is used to lull the patient into relaxation.

46. T   F   The patient with peripheral vascular disease should not wear circular garters.

47. T   F   The safest way to supply warmth to a patient with peripheral vascular disease is to apply a heating pad.

48. T   F   People with poor peripheral circulation should be encouraged to smoke.

49. T   F   In atherosclerosis blood vessels become widely dilated.

50. T   F   Severe crushing chest pain may be a symptom of an MI.

51. T   F   Heart failure is also known as PVD.

52. T   F   The anemic patient may require special mouth care.

53. T   F   The anemic person is pale and may experience exhaustion and dyspnea.

54. T   F   Sickle cell anemia is due to an inability to absorb vitamin B12.

55. T   F   The nursing care of the person with leukemia is similar to that given to the person with anemia.

Clinical Situations. Briefly describe how a nursing assistant should react to the following situations.

56. Your patient, who has angina pectoris, is having an argument with a visitor.

_____

_____

57. You are passing out trays and find a salt shaker on the tray of your patient with congestive heart failure.

_____

58. The patient with congestive heart failure has an erratic radial pulse rate of 72.

_____

59. The patient with congestive heart failure has a fluid intake far in excess of output.

_____

60. Your patient who has hypertension suddenly complains of blurred vision and his speech is slurred. _____

_____

RELATING TO THE NURSING PROCESS

Write the step of the nursing process that is related to the nursing assistant action.

Nursing Assistant Action   **Nursing Process Step**

61. The nursing assistant reports that the resident's legs are pale in color and cool in touch.

_____

62. The nursing assistant daily weighs the patient suffering with congestive heart failure.

_____

63. The nursing assistant completes the bath for the patient with congestive heart failure to lessen fatigue.

_____

64. The nursing assistant provides special mouth care for the patient with anemia.

_____

65. The nursing assistant reports that the patient who is anemic tires very easily.

_____

DEVELOPING GREATER INSIGHT

66. Think through reasons why properly fitting shoes should be worn by the patient with peripheral vascular disease when out of bed.

67. Discuss with classmates the kinds of concerns you might have if you were dependent on a pacemaker.

68. Practice finding and measuring the pulse in each of the followint vessels:

    a. temporal

    b. carotid

    c. popliteal

    d. dorsalis pedis

69. Think through why people who cross their legs, sit long hours at work, or have the heavy weight of pregnancy in the abdomen tend to develop varicose veins.

UNIT 38   Musculoskeletal System

OBJECTIVES

As a result of this unit, you will be able to:

- Spell and define terms.

- Describe the location and functions of the musculoskeletal system.

- Describe some common conditions of the musculoskeletal system.

- Describe the nursing assistant actions related to the care of patients with conditions and diseases of the musculoskeletal system.

- List seven specific diagnostic tests for musculoskeletal conditions.

- Demonstrate the following procedure:

Procedure 94 Performing Range-of-Motion Exercises (Passive)

UNIT SUMMARY

- Orthopedic injuries often require long periods of immobilization and rehabilitation.

- Routine range-of-motion exercises must be carried out for all uninjured joints to:

Prevent deformities and joint stiffening.
Promote general circulation.
Prevent mineral loss from the bones.

- Special nursing care for patients in casts and traction or with a hip prosthesis:

Ensures proper alignment.
Prevents pressure areas.
Avoids skin breakdown.

NURSING ASSISTANT ALERT

Action	Benefit
Encourage activity that is consistent with individual patient limitations.	Prevents loss of mobility. Limits the development of contractures.
Maintain and promote proper alignment.	Encourages optimum functional ability.
Carry out range of motion for those patients unable to assist themselves.	Maintains mobility and prevents contractures.

ACTIVITIES

Vocabulary Exercise. Each line has four different spellings of a word. Circle the correctly spelled word.

1. barsitis	bursitis	bursites	buresitis
2. cartilage	cartalage	cartilege	catelage
3. comminnuted	cominuted	comminooted	comminuted
4. suppinachon	suppination	supination	suppinasion
5. virtebrae	vertabrae	vertebrae	vertobrae
6. extension	extinsion	extenchon	extention
7. aduction	adducsion	adduchon	adduction
8. dorsiflexion	dorseflexion	dorsiflextion	dorsifection

Anatomy Review. Using colored pencils or crayons, color in the following bones as indicated.

9. a. femur—red

   b. humerus—blue

   c. ribs—brown

   d. ulna—green

   e. radius—red

   f. sternum—brown

   g. pelvis—blue

   h. cranium—green

   i. tibia—yellow

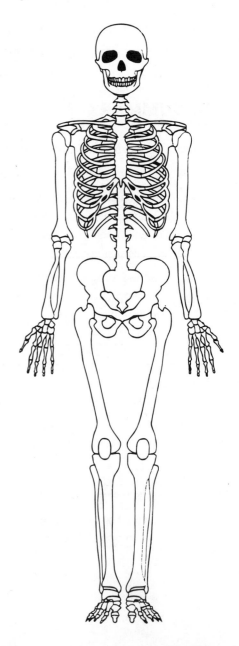

Completion. Complete the statements in the spaces provided.

10. To remain healthy, the musculoskeletal system must be _____.

11. Abnormal shortening of muscles is called _____.

12. Moving each toe away from the second toe is called _____.

13. Moving each finger toward the middle finger is called _____.

14. Touching the thumb to the little finger of the same hand is called _____.

15. Rolling the hip in a circular motion toward the midline is called _____.

16. Small fluid-filled sacs found around joints are called _____.

17. Inflammation of a joint is called _____.

18. Any break in the continuity of a bone is a _____.

19. If the broken bone protrudes through the skin, it is called a _____ fracture.

20. Traction that uses several weights and lines is called _____ traction.

Brief Answers. Briefly answer the following questions.

21. What are four dangers of insufficient exercise?

    a. _____

    b. _____

    c. _____

    d. _____

22. What five special techniques should you use when carrying out ROM exercises?

    a. _____

    b. _____

    c. _____

    d. _____

23. What five techniques are used to treat chronic arthritis?

    a. _____

    b. _____

    c. _____

    d. _____

24. What are five ways to immobilize a fracture?

    a. _____

    b. _____

    c. _____

    d. _____

25. What two special beds are sometimes used when patients have multiple fractures?

    a. _____

    b. _____

26. What eight special nursing care procedures must be given to the patient in a fresh leg cast?

    a. _____

b. _____

c. _____

d. _____

e. _____

f. _____

g. _____

h. _____

27. What are four general factors to keep in mind as care is given to the patient in traction?

a. _____

b. _____

c. _____

d. _____

28. Define the following range-of-motion terms:

a. extension _____

b. abduction _____

c. rotation: lateral _____

d. eversion _____

e. inversion _____

f. pronation _____

g. radial deviation _____

h. ulnar deviation _____

i. plantar flexion _____

j. dorsiflexion _____

29. Identify the fractures by writing the proper names in the spaces provided.

a. _____   b. _____   c. _____   d. _____

a.   b.   c.   d.

30. Contrast two forms of chronic arthritis.

Form	Tissue Affected	Possible Cause	Age Affected
Rheumatoid Arthritis			
Osteoarthritis			

31. Identify the traction lines using colored pencils. Follow the directions.

    Figure A: With a red pencil, color the traction belt and trace the primary pelvic traction lines.

    Figure B: With a red pencil, trace the primary cervical traction line.

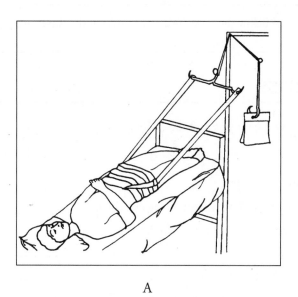

A

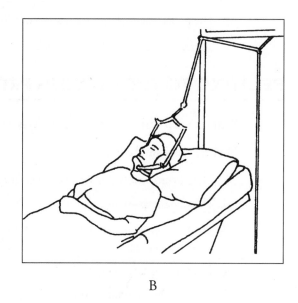

B

32. Figures A and B represent two patients who each have a new right hip prosthesis. Identify the incorrect behavior being demonstrated.

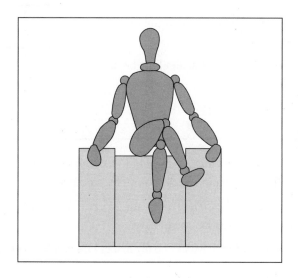

A

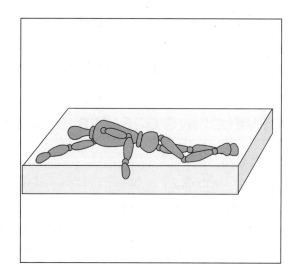

B

Clinical Situations. Briefly describe how a nursing assistant should react to the following situations.

33. The toes of your patient in a leg cast felt cold and looked bluish. _____

_____

34. You found that your patient in pelvic traction had the feet pressed against the foot of the bed.

_____

_____

35. Your patient complained of discomfort during range-of-motion exercises. _____

_____

36. The patient's traction is to be discontinued. _____

_____

37. The patient has had an amputation of a lower leg below the knee. You must position the extremity. _____

_____

RELATING TO THE NURSING PROCESS

Write the step of the nursing process that is related to the nursing assistant action.

Nursing Assistant Action	Nursing Process Step
38. The nursing assistant handles the wet cast with open palms.	_____
39. The nursing assistant supports each joint above and below the joint being exercised.	_____
40. The nursing assistant stops carrying out range of motion and reports to the nurse when the patient complains of pain.	_____
41. The nursing assistant carries out each ROM exercise five times.	_____
42. The nursing assistant reports the patient's feelings of numbness in the toes of the newly casted leg.	_____
43. The nursing assistant helps support the patient in a spica cast while another assistant changes the linen.	_____
44. The nursing assistant is very careful not to disturb the weights while caring for the patient in traction.	_____
45. The nursing assistant asks the nursing supervisor to review the traction lines before she begins to give care.	_____

DEVELOPING GREATER INSIGHT

46. Stand in front of a full-length mirror. Be sure you have something to hang onto for support. Raise one leg, bending it at the knee, and pretend you have had an amputation. How do you feel about your body image now?

47. Wrap one leg in an Ace Bandage so you will keep your knee straight, simulating a cast. Try to ambulate safely using crutches. Identify difficulties a patient in a similar situation might have.

48. Put your dominant arm in a sling and try to carry out your activities of daily living. Did you feel frustrated by the experience?

49. Working in pairs, take turns being patient and nursing assistant and practice passive ROM exercises.

UNIT 39   Endocrine System

OBJECTIVES

As a result of this unit, you will be able to:

- Spell and define terms.

- Review the location and functions of the endocrine system.

- List five specific diagnostic tests associated with conditions of the endocrine system.

- Describe some common diseases of the endocrine system.

- Recognize the signs and symptoms of hypoglycemia and hyperglycemia.

- Describe nursing assistant actions related to the care of patients with disorders of the endocrine system.

- Perform blood tests for glucose levels if facility policy permits.

- Perform the following procedures:

    Procedure 95 Testing Urine for Acetone: Ketostix® Strip Test

UNIT SUMMARY

- Endocrine glands:

- Secrete hormones that influence body activities.

- Are subject to disease and malfunction.

Common conditions of the endocrine system are those involving:
- The thyroid gland. These are hyperthyroidism or hypothyroidism.

- The pancreas. A major condition is diabetes mellitus.

Diabetes mellitus:
- Affects many people.

- May be treated with a balance of:

    Diet.
    Exercise.
    Hypoglycemic drugs or insulin.
- Requires conscientious nursing care to avoid serious complications.

- Requires understanding by the patient of the need to follow the therapeutic program.

NURSING ASSISTANT ALERT

Action	Benefit
Know the signs and symptoms of impending diabetic coma and insulin shock and report at once.	Early intervention can prevent development of serious complications.

Action	Benefit
Give special attention to the diabetic's feet and dietary intake.	Contributes to foot health and proper blood sugar levels.
Follow orders faithfully and report response.	Helps those who are hormonally imbalanced to be stabilized.

ACTIVITIES

Vocabulary Exercise. Complete the puzzle by filling in the missing letters of words found in this unit. Use the definitions to help you discover these words.

1. __ __ __ __ __ __ E   1. blood sugar
2. __ __ __ __ __ N __   2. endocrine secretion
3. __ __ __ __ __ D __ __ __   3. being diseased
4. __ __ __ __ O __ __ __ __   4. produced by thyroid gland
5. __ __ __ C __ __ __ __ __ __ 5. sugar in the urine
6. R   6.
7. __ __ __ I __ __   7. needed for production of thyroxine
8. __ __ __ N __ __   8. organs that secrete body fluids
9. __ __ E __ __   9. male reproductive cell

Definitions. Define the following terms or abbreviations in the spaces provided.

10. BMR _____

11. hypersecretion _____

12. hypertrophy _____

13. mortality rate _____

14. polydipsia _____

15. tetany _____

Anatomy Review. Using colored pencils, color the glands as indicated.

16. ovaries—red

17. thyroid—green

18. pituitary—blue

19. parathyroids—black

20. adrenals—brown

21. pancreas—red

22. pineal body—green

23. testes—yellow

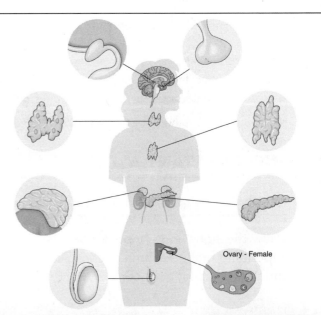

Ovary - Female

Completion. Complete the following statements in the spaces provided.

24. The role of glands in the body is to secrete _____.

25. The chemicals secreted by glands _____ body activities and growth.

26. A major contribution the nursing assistant can make to the care of a patient with hyperthyroidism is to keep the room _____ and be patient and calm.

27. The treatment for hyperthyroidism is to _____ the level of thyroxine production.

28. Hypothyroidism can occur even when the thyroid gland _____.

29. The role of parathormone is to regulate the electrolyte levels of _____ and _____.

30. One of the severe effects of inadequate levels of parathormone is severe muscle spasm called _____.

31. Hypersecretion of adrenal cortical hormones causes a disease syndrome called _____.

32. The patient with Addison's disease becomes dehydrated and has a low tolerance to _____.

33. The diabetic exchange system was formulated by a committee with representatives from the _____ and the diabetes branch of the _____.

34. Measurement of foods in the exchange system is based on standard _____ measurements.

35. Beside diet and insulin, another important part of diabetic therapy is _____.

36. Two medications given in diabetes mellitus are insulin and _____ drugs.

37. The patient with diabetes has a sweet, fruity odor to his breath, so you might suspect _____.

38. The patient with diabetes is feeling excited, nervous, and hungry, so you might suspect _____.

39. All urine being tested for acetone must be _____ voided.

40. Daily foot care for the diabetic includes washing, drying, and _____ the feet.

41. Toenails of the diabetic should be cut only by a _____.

42. Diabetic patients should never be permitted to go _____.

43. The radioactive iodine uptake test is performed to check _____.

44. Special care must be taken of the _____ of the patient with diabetes.

Brief Answers Briefly answer the following questions.

45. How might the person with hyperthyroidism look and behave?

_____

_____

46. Your patient has just returned from surgery following a partial thyroidectomy. What should you check for and report?

a. _____

b. _____

c. _____

d. _____

e. _____

f. _____

47. What happens to the patient who develops hypersecretion of the parathyroid gland?

    a. _____

    b. _____

    c. _____

48. How might Cushing's syndrome be demonstrated in the female patient?

    a. _____

    b. _____

    c. _____

    d. _____

    e. _____

    f. _____

49. What three factors seem to play a role in the incidence of diabetes mellitus?

    a. _____

    b. _____

    c. _____

50. What complications are common to the patient who suffers uncontrolled diabetes mellitus for many years?

    a. _____

    b. _____

    c. _____

    d. _____

    e. _____

    f. _____

51. What role does diet play in the care of the diabetic patient?

    _____

52. What five factors can contribute to a hyperglycemic state?

    a. _____

    b. _____

    c. _____

    d. _____

    e. _____

53. What six factors can contribute to a hypoglycemic state?

    a. _____

    b. _____

    c. _____

    d. _____

    e. _____

    f. _____

54. What are ten nursing assistant responsibilities in caring for the insulin-dependent diabetes mellitus patient?

a. _____

b. _____

c. _____

d. _____

e. _____

f. _____

g. _____

h. _____

i. _____

j. _____

55. Which five metabolic functions are upset when there is insufficient insulin?

a. _____

b. _____

c. _____

d. _____

e. _____

56. What are the typical signs and symptoms associated with IDDM diabetes mellitus?

a. _____

b. _____

c. _____

d. _____

57. For what do the abbreviations stand?

a. IDDM _____

b. NIDDM _____

58. What care should be given to the feet of the patient with diabetes?

a. _____   d. _____

b. _____   e. _____

c. _____   f. _____

59. Compare the signs and symptoms of diabetic coma and insulin shock.

	Diabetic Coma	Insulin Shock
Respirations		
Pulse		
Skin		

Clinical Situations. Briefly describe how a nursing assistant should react to the following situations.

60. Your patient is to have a BMR at 8 A.M. _____

_____

_____

_____

61. Your older obese patient complains of constant fatigue and burning on urination. She has a bruise on her leg that is healing poorly. _____

_____

_____

62. Your postoperative thyroidectomy patient has increasing difficulty speaking. _____

_____

63. Your postoperative thyroidectomy patient has moved down in the bed so that the neck is hyperextended.

_____

_____

RELATING TO THE NURSING PROCESS

Write the step of the nursing process that is related to the nursing assistant action.

Nursing Assistant Action	Nursing Process Step
64. The nursing assistant reports that her patient, a diabetic, has diarrhea.	_____
65. The nursing assistant makes sure the room of the patient with hyperthyroidism is kept cool and quiet.	_____
66. The nursing assistant documents the amount of fluid the patient with diabetes is consuming.	_____
67. The nursing assistant reports that the patient with diabetes has pale, moist skin and seems nervous.	_____
68. The nursing assistant tests the patient's urine for acetone using the Ketostix® strip test.	_____
69. The nursing assistant carefully washes and inspects the feet of the patient with diabetes daily.	_____

DEVELOPING GREATER INSIGHT

70. Make a list of ways your life would change if you were diagnosed with diabetes mellitus type II. Share your list with the class.

71. Test your own urine for acetone using a Ketostix® strip tape.

UNIT 40   Nervous System

OBJECTIVES

As a result of this unit, you will be able to:

- Spell and define terms.

- State the location and functions of the organs of the nervous system.

- List five diagnostic tests used to determine conditions of the nervous system.

- Describe eight common conditions of the nervous system.

- Describe nursing assistant actions related to the care of patients with conditions of the nervous system.

- Explain the proper care, handling, and insertion of an artificial eye.

- Explain the proper care, handling, and insertion of a hearing aid.

- Demonstrate the following procedures:

    Procedure 96 Caring for Eye Socket and Artificial Eye
    Procedure 97 Applying a Behind-the-Ear Hearing Aid
    Procedure 98 Removing a Behind-the-Ear Hearing Aid
    Procedure 99 Applying and Removing an In-the-Ear Hearing Aid

UNIT SUMMARY

The nursing assistant assists the professional nurse in the care of patients with neurological conditions. Although the professional nurse is responsible for neurological assessment and intervention, the alert nursing assistant can make valuable observations.

- Observations of changes in levels of consciousness, response, and behavior must be accurately and promptly reported.

- The nursing assistant supplies comfort and support during the critical care period.

- Under supervision, the nursing assistant provides specific care for patients who have the following conditions:

    CVAs
    Seizures
    Head injuries
    Spinal cord injuries
    Diseases of or trauma to the eyes and ears

Diseases and injuries of the nervous system often require a long recovery period. During the convalescent period, the nursing assistant plays an important role. Patience, empathy, and skill are needed in full measure to assist these patients in their recovery.

NURSING ASSISTANT ALERT

Action	Benefit
Document observations and care accurately.	Provides a database for correct nursing evaluations and interventions.
Patiently use a variety of communication skills.	Lessens patient frustration. Improves accuracy of messages sent and received.
Be consistent in care and use established routines	Requires fewer stressful adjustments for the patient.

ACTIVITIES

Vocabulary Exercise. Complete the crossword puzzle by using the definitions provided.

Down

1. chemical needed for nerve transmission
2. bundle of nerve processes
3. portion of neuron that carries the impulse of the cell
4. organ of hearing in inner ear

Across

5. within the skull
6. part of eye in front of lens
7. loss of motor control in all four limbs
8. trembling

Definitions. Define the following terms or abbreviations in the spaces provided.

9. akinesia _____

10. ossicles _____

11. aphasia _____

12. meninges _____

13. tremors _____

14. paralysis _____

15. Lhermitte's sign _____

16. quadriplegia _____

17. nystagmus _____

18. convulsion _____

Anatomy Review. Using colored pencils, or crayons, color the functional areas of the brain as indicated.

19. movement—red

20. hearing—yellow

21. pain and other sensations—green

22. seeing—brown

23. speech and language—blue

24. spinal cord—black

Completion. Complete the following statements in the spaces provided.

25. The pressure of tissue and fluid within the skull is called _____ pressure.

26. Other names for stroke are _____ or cerebrovascular accident.

27. The symptoms of a brain attack depend on the area of _____ that becomes ischemic.

28. Left brain damage often results in loss of _____.

29. Post-stroke patients have a high level of _____.

30. TIAs are sometimes called _____.

31. The incidence of macular degeneration increases with _____.

32. Following cataract surgery, the patient should avoid _____.

33. Following cataract surgery, it is especially important to report _____ in the operative eye.

34. Otitis media is an infection of the _____ and may result in _____ of the ossicles leading to deafness.

35. It is important not to let a hearing aid get _____.

Brief Answers.   Briefly answer the following questions.

36. What are six signs that the intracranial pressure is rising in a patient with a head injury?

a. _____

b. _____

c. _____

d. _____

e. _____

f. _____

37. What seven changes in the patient with a brain injury must be noted and reported to the nurse?

a. _____

b. _____

c. _____

d. _____

e. _____

f. _____

g. _____

38. What are seven nursing care measures that must be maintained throughout the acute and convalescent care of a person with a head injury?

a. _____

b. _____

c. _____

d. _____

e. _____

f. _____

g. _____

39. What four ways can the nursing assistant help the aphasic patient communicate?

a. _____

b. _____

c. _____

d. _____

40. What eight nursing care measures must be carried out when caring for the patient in the acute phase of a cerebrovascular accident?

a. _____

b. _____

c. _____

d. _____

e. _____

f. _____

g. _____

h. _____

41. What are two important goals of nursing care of a patient during a seizure?

a. _____

b. _____

42. What are three ways to prevent contractures in the patient with a spinal cord injury?

a. _____

b. _____

c. _____

43. What are two positions in which spinal punctures are usually performed?

a. _____

b. _____

44. What two techniques can be learned to help communicate with someone who is deaf?

a. _____

b. _____

45. Complete the chart.

Type of Seizure	Description
a. petit mal	
b. grand mal	
c. status epilepticus	

True/False. Mark the following true or false by circling T or F.

46. T F   Patients who are paralyzed are prone to pressure ulcers.

47. T F   The ear mold of a hearing aid is removed by lifting the mold upward and outward.

48. T F   During a seizure, an airway is best maintained by keeping the head straight.

49. T F   Parkinson's disease is characterized by muscular rigidity and akinesia.

50. T F   Intention tremors become worse as the individual tries to touch or pick up an object.

51. T F   Multiple sclerosis is a progressive disease associated with inadequate levels of neuro-transmitters in the cerebellum and brain stem.

52. T F   Seizure syndrome is sometimes known as epilepsy.

53. T F   Patients with spinal cord injuries need long-term nursing care.

54. T F   Meningitis is an inflammation of the inner ear resulting in deafness.

Clinical Situations. Briefly describe how a nursing assistant should react to the following situations.

55. The patient is on the floor convulsing. _____

_____

56. You notice a change in the level of consciousness of your patient with a head injury.

_____

_____

_____

57. The patient is very hard of hearing and wears a hearing aid.

   a. _____

   b. _____

   c. _____

   d. _____

   e. _____

   f. _____

   g. _____

   h. _____

   i. _____

RELATING TO THE NURSING PROCESS

Write the step of the nursing process that is related to the nursing assistant action.

Nursing Assistant Action	**Nursing Process Step**
58. The nursing assistant notes uncontrolled body movements in the patient with a head injury and calls this to the nurse's attention.	_____
59. The nursing assistant helps the nurse turn and position the patient suffering from a stroke.	_____
60. The nursing assistant carries out ROM exercises for the patient who is paralyzed.	_____
61. The nursing assistant finds a patient who is convulsing. She calls for help but does not leave the patient alone.	_____
62. The nursing assistant uses a picture board to assist communication with a patient who has aphasia.	_____
63. The nursing assistant pays particular attention when the patient with Parkinson's disease ambulates, knowing that he is more apt to fall.	_____
64. The nursing assistant and all staff members try to maintain a calm environment for the patients with Parkinson's disease.	_____

DEVELOPING GREATER INSIGHT

65. Put cotton balls in your ears and try to communicate with your classmates. Discuss your feelings and frustrations.

66. Try communicating your feelings and needs to a classmate without words and without the use of one hand and arm. Describe your feelings.

UNIT 41   Gastrointestinal System

OBJECTIVES

As a result of this unit, you will be able to:

- Spell and define terms.

- Review the location and functions of the organs of the gastrointestinal system.

- List specific diagnostic tests associated with disorders of the gastrointestinal system.

- Describe some common disorders of the gastrointestinal system.

- Describe nursing assistant actions related to the care of patients with disorders of the gastrointestinal system.

- Identify different types of enemas and state their purpose.

- Demonstrate the following procedures:

  Procedure 100 Collecting a Stool Specimen
  Procedure 101 Giving a Soap Solution Enema
  Procedure 102 Giving a Commercially Prepared Enema
  Procedure 103 Inserting a Rectal Suppository
  Procedure 104 Inserting a Rectal Tube and Flatus Bag

UNIT SUMMARY

- The organs in the digestive system are very complex. Because of their complexity, disease of these organs is fairly common. Common conditions include:

  - Cancer   - Hernias
  - Ulcerations   - Inflammation such as cholecystitis

- Procedures performed on this system include:

  Enemas. Enemas are also performed before surgery on other parts of the body.
  Insertion of rectal tubes to relieve flatus.
  Insertion of rectal suppositories.

- Great care must be exercised when performing the procedures. Remember that the comfort and privacy of the patient should be protected at all times.

NURSING ASSISTANT ALERT

Action	Benefit
Provide adequate coverage and privacy.	Diminishes patient anxiety and embarrassment.
Maintain a matter-of-fact attitude.	Protects patient's self-esteem.
Prepare patients for tests according to orders	Ensures more successful testing.

ACTIVITIES

Vocabulary Exercise. Put a circle around the word defined.

1. removal of a gall bladder
2. removal of the stomach
3. artificial opening made in the large bowel for fecal elimination
4. eliminating feces through the anus
5. another name for the large bowel
6. protrusion of the intestines through a weakened area in the abdominal wall
7. collection of hardened feces in the rectum
8. intestinal gas
9. a strong feeling of the need to eliminate
10. pertaining to the stomach

```
X A D E F E C A T I O N J L
S G N B M R I Y P T Z G T D
V A C U O N P E N C R A Q L
G S K T R Z F M L Y E S W U
E T V E R C L H M X O T M R
P R H Q X L A O K T X R O G
J I M P A C T I O N D E A E
F C O N E S U Y S R T C M N
S F L O O P S E J M Q T S C
C H O L E C Y S T E T O M Y
P S O K L T Z Y E N Y M E S
D C N U V C O L O N D Y F P
```

Definitions. Define the following terms or abbreviations.

11. HCl _____

12. cholelithiasis _____

13. peristalsis _____

14. herniorrhaphy _____

15. impaction _____

16. gavage _____

17. duodenum _____

18. inguinal _____

19. incarcerated _____

20. TWE _____

Anatomy Review. Using colored pencils, or crayons, color the organs of the digestive system as indicated.

21. esophagus—blue

22. stomach—yellow

23. small intestine—green

24. liver—red

25. gallbladder—black

26. colon—blue

27. appendix—brown

28. pancreas—blue

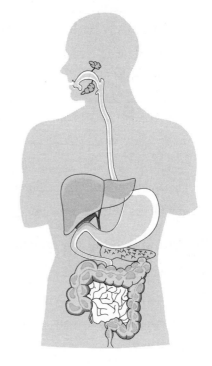

Completion. Complete the following statements in the spaces provided.

29. A common condition affecting the gastrointestinal tract is _____, which can often cause obstructions.

30. If a patient has a nasogastric tube in place, you must be very careful not to allow anything to _____.

31. Following a bowel resection, it may be necessary to create an artificial opening called a _____.

32. The patient with ulcerative colitis becomes dehydrated because of frequent _____.

33. The patient with ulcerative colitis should be eating a high-protein, high-calorie, _____ diet.

34. The patient with a duodenal ulcer is given medication to neutralize the _____ of the stomach, which causes additional trauma to the _____ area.

35. If a patient is placed on NPO, special _____ should be given.

36. The patient with cholecystitis or cholelithiasis is usually placed on a low-_____ diet.

37. Following a cholecystectomy, _____ are often placed in the operative area.

38. In addition to routine postoperative care, the cholecystectomy patient should be placed in the _____ position.

39. Your patient is scheduled for a GB series, so you should check for orders regarding _____ or a special _____.

40. The solution used for a soap solution enema is _____.

41. The best patient position for administration of an enema is the _____.

42. When possible, an enema should be given _____ giving the bath.

43. A _____ is required before giving an enema.

44. An oil retention enema is retained and followed with a _____ enema.

45. The lubricated enema tube should be inserted _____ into the anus.

46. The enema solution container should be raised _____ above the level of the _____ while allowing the fluid to flow into the patient.

47. Reusable enema equipment should be rinsed in _____ water before washing.

48. The rectal tube is used to relieve abdominal _____.

49. Commercially prepared chemical enema solutions drain fluid from the body to stimulate _____.

50. The chemical enema solution should be retained as _____.

51. Rectal tubes should be used no more than _____ in 24 hours.

52. Standard precautions require the use of _____ to protect the _____ from contamination during procedures involving the anus or rectum.

53. Antibiotics are given to control _____ that is involved in the development of gastric ulcers.

Brief Answers Briefly answer the following questions.

54. Symptoms that might indicate a bowel malignancy include:

    a. _____

    b. _____

    c. _____

    d. _____

    e. _____

    f. _____

55. What are three important observations regarding your patient who has had a cholecystectomy that should immediately be reported to your team leader?

    a. _____

    b. _____

    c. _____

56. What are five reasons that enemas are commonly given?

    a. _____

    b. _____

    c. _____

    d. _____

    e. _____

57. What information should be included in documenting an enema?

    a. _____

    b. _____

    c. _____

    d. _____

58. What are four sites where hernias frequently develop?

    a. _____

    b. _____

    c. _____

    d. _____

Clinical Situations. Briefly describe how a nursing assistant should react to the following situations.

59. You have an order to give a soap solution enema and the patient has just finished breakfast.

_____

60. The patient complains of cramping while you are giving an enema.

_____

61. Your patient has returned from surgery following a cholecystectomy. Drains are in place.

_____

62. Your patient expresses concern about retaining a rectal suppository.

_____

RELATING TO THE NURSING PROCESS

Write the step of the nursing process that is related to the nursing assistant action.

Nursing Assistant Action	Nursing Process Step
63. The nursing assistant carefully explains the procedure before administering an enema to the patient.	_____
64. The nursing assistant inserts a lubricating suppository beyond the rectal sphincter.	_____
65. The nursing assistant instructs the patient that an oil retention enema must be retained for at least 20 minutes after introduction.	_____
66. The nursing assistant lubricates the tip of the enema tube well before insertion.	_____
67. The nursing assistant reports and records the results of the soap solution enema.	_____

DEVELOPING GREATER INSIGHT

68. Tumors of the colon can often grow large before being detected. Can you think why this might be? _____

_____

69. Discuss reasons why enemas are given before a meal rather than after. _____

_____

UNIT 42   Urinary System

OBJECTIVES

As a result of this unit, you will be able to:
■ Spell and define terms.

■ Review the location and function of the urinary system.

■ List five diagnostic tests associated with conditions of the urinary system.

■ Describe some common diseases of the urinary system.

■ Describe nursing assistant actions related to the care of patients with urinary system diseases and conditions.

Procedure 105 Collecting a Routine Urine Specimen
Procedure 106 Collecting a Clean-Catch Urine Specimen
Procedure 107 Collecting a Fresh Fractional Urine Specimen
Procedure 108 Collecting a 24-Hour Urine Specimen
Procedure 109 Testing Urine with the HemaCombistix®
Procedure 110 Routine Drainage Check
Procedure 111 Giving Indwelling Catheter Care
Procedure 112 Emptying a Urinary Drainage Unit
Procedure 113 Disconnecting the Catheter
Procedure 114 Replacing a Condom for Urinary Drainage
Procedure 115 Connecting a Catheter to a Leg Bag
Procedure 116 Emptying a Leg Bag

UNIT SUMMARY

Two vital nursing measures necessary in the care of patients with urinary dysfunction are:
■ Maintaining adequate urinary drainage.

■ Keeping drainage equipment free of contamination.

The urinary track is considered a sterile area. Special sterile techniques must be used when the physician or nurse introduces a catheter into this area. The nursing assistant must know how to safely:
■ Disconnect the catheter from the drainage setup.

■ Empty and measure the drainage.

■ Ambulate the patient with constant urinary drainage.

NURSING ASSISTANT ALERT

Action	Benefit
Secure and care for urine specimens according to policy.	Contributes to more accurate data.
Maintain patency in the urinary drainage system.	Prevents backup of urine and subsequent damage.
Maintain accurate I&O records	Helps to monitor renal function.
Protect drainage tubing connection site.	Keeps drainage system free from contamination.
Keep drainage bag below level of bladder.	Prevents reflux of drained urine into the bladder.

ACTIVITIES

Vocabulary Exercise. Unscramble the words introduced in this unit and define them.

1. YSIDURA _____

2. HAEUMRTAI _____

3. RODSHIYSNPEHOR _____

4. NIKEDYS _____

5. RTIENNOTE _____

6. EEURRT _____

7. HPREINTSI _____

8. TISTCYIS _____

9. MULOLGIER _____

Definitions. Define the terms or abbreviations.

10. oliguria _____

11. renal calculi _____

12. IVP _____

13. suppression _____

14. catheter _____

15. meatus _____

Anatomy Review. Using colored pencils, or crayons, color the organs of the urinary system as indicated.

16. right kidney—red

17. ureters—blue

18. bladder—green

19. urethra—yellow

20. adrenal glands—brown

21. left kidney cortex—red

22. left kidney medulla—blue

23. left kidney pelvis—yellow

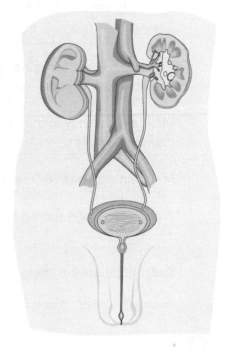

Completion. Complete the following statements in the spaces provided.

24. Cystitis is a fairly common problem in _____ because of the shortness of the urethra.

25. Patients with cystitis may find relief from a bladder spasm using a _____ bath.

26. Fluid intake should be _____ in cystitis patients.

27. You might expect the blood pressure of a patient with long-standing renal disease to be _____.

28. Edema is common in nephritis because of diminished ability of the kidneys to _____.

29. Renal calculi can cause _____ to the normal flow of urine.

30. The sudden intense pain associated with renal calculi is known as renal _____.

31. Because of the damage done by renal calculi, blood in the urine is common. This is known as _____.

32. All the urine of a patient with renal calculi should be _____.

33. The patient with renal calculi should have fluids _____.

34. Lithotripsy is a technique used to _____ renal calculi.

35. Destructive accumulation of fluid in the kidney is called _____.

36. The Foley catheter has a _____ surrounding the neck so it can be retained in the bladder.

37. The insertion of a catheter is a _____ procedure and should be performed by the _____ or _____.

38. Urinary condoms can be used on _____ patients needing long-term drainage.

39. It is _____ never to disconnect the drainage setup, but it may be necessary.

40. Special care is needed when there are urinary conditions because the urinary tract is considered to be a _____ area.

41. Properties of a fresh urine specimen begin to be altered after _____ minutes.

42. If a sample of urine cannot be delivered to the laboratory immediately, it should be _____.

43. Approximately _____ of urine are sent to the laboratory as a specimen.

44. Before collecting a midstream urine specimen, always clean the area around the _____ and then allow some urine to be expelled.

45. The 24-hour urine specimen requires that the patient start the 24-hour interval with the bladder _____.

46. The last urine voided is _____ in the 24-hour specimen.

Brief Answers. Briefly answer the following questions.

47. How might a person demonstrate the signs and symptoms of cystitis?

    a. _____
    b. _____
    c. _____
    d. _____

48. What orders might be written for the patient with severe nephritis?

    a. _____
    b. _____
    c. _____
    d. _____

49. What important nursing procedures must the nursing assistant carry out following removal of renal calculi?

    _____

    _____

50. Besides carefully reporting I&O, what other signs and symptoms should immediately be reported in a patient following a nephrectomy?

    a. _____
    b. _____
    c. _____
    d. _____
    e. _____
    f. _____

51. What are two common types of catheters used to drain the urinary bladder?

    a. _____
    b. _____

52. What are seven responsibilities the nursing assistant has when caring for a patient with urinary drainage?

    a. _____
    b. _____
    c. _____
    d. _____
    e. _____
    f. _____
    g. _____

53. If urinary drainage must be disconnected, what parts must be protected against contamination?

    a. _____
    b. _____

Clinical Situations. Briefly describe how a nursing assistant should react to the following situations.

54. Your patient has an indwelling catheter. Explain the daily care you will provide. _____

_____

_____

55. Your patient has condom drainage. List three responsibilities of the nursing assistant. _____

_____

_____

56. Your patient is on I&O. Explain how to measure the drainage when the patient has an indwelling catheter. _____

_____

_____

57. Your patient has urinary drainage into a leg bag. List four points to keep in mind while providing care.

a. _____

b. _____

c. _____

d. _____

RELATING TO THE NURSING PROCESS

Write the step of the nursing process that is related to the nursing assistant action.

Nursing Assistant Action	Nursing Process Step
58. The nursing assistant promptly reports that the patient is experiencing chills.	_____
59. The nursing assistant checks the drainage tubing to be sure it is taped properly.	_____
60. The nursing assistant is careful not to let the tip of the urine drainage tube touch the side of the graduate when the bag is emptied.	_____
61. The nursing assistant wears gloves when handling the patient's urinary drainage equipment.	_____
62. The nursing assistant strains all urine as ordered when the patient has renal calculi.	_____
63. If the patient is not circumcised, the nursing assistant makes sure to reposition the foreskin after giving indwelling catheter care.	_____
64. The nursing assistant maintains a positive attitude when changing the soiled linen of a patient who is incontinent.	_____
65. The nursing assistant uses standard precautions to collect and measure a urine specimen.	_____
66. All the nursing assistants add urine to a 24-hour collection from a single patient even though the patient is the primary responsibility of one nursing assistant.	_____

DEVELOPING GREATER INSIGHT

67. Discuss with classmates why continence is so important to self-esteem.

68. Discuss with classmates why gloves are to be worn when handling bedpans or urine samples.

UNIT 43   Reproductive System

OBJECTIVES

As a result of this unit, you will be able to:

- Spell and define terms.

- Review the location and functions of the organs of the male and female reproductive systems.

- List six diagnostic tests associated with conditions of the male and female reproductive systems.

- Describe some common disorders and conditions of the male reproductive system.

- Describe some common disorders and conditions of the female reproductive system.

- Describe nursing assistant actions related to the care of patients with conditions and diseases of the reproductive system.

- State the nursing precautions required for patients who have sexually transmitted diseases.

- Demonstrate the following procedures:

  Procedure 117 Breast Self-Examination
  Procedure 118 Giving a Nonsterile Vaginal Douche

UNIT SUMMARY

- A knowledge of the normal male and female reproductive structures is important for the nursing assistant who wishes to understand the related nursing care.

- Disposable equipment available in many hospitals makes nursing care more convenient and safer for the patient.

- The nursing assistant must be understanding and patient when providing care for patients with reproductive problems, because any surgery on the reproductive organs may have a strong psychological effect on the patient.

- The nursing assistant must practice proper infection control when caring for patients with sexually transmitted diseases.

NURSING ASSISTANT ALERT

Action	Benefit
Be alert to and report indications of infections or abnormalities of the reproductive tract.	Therapy can be started early that can avert more extensive body damage.
Practice breast or testicular self-examination regularly.	Protects your own health.
Remember there is a strong relationship between the reproductive system and sexual identity.	Contributes to accepting the individual as a sexual being.

Action	Benefit
Recognize that any threat to the reproductive organs has a strong psychological impact on an individual.	Allows staff to be supportive.

ACTIVITIES

Vocabulary Exercise. Complete the puzzle by filling in the missing letters of words found in this unit. Use the definitions to help you discover these words.

1. — — — — M — — — — — —   1. lining of the uterus
2. — — — — — E — —   2. protrusion of rectum into vagina
3.   N   3.
4. — — S — — — — — —   4. excision of a breast
5. — — T — —   5. male sex glands
6. — — R — —   6. womb
7. — — — U — —   7. term for fallopian tube
8. — A — — —   8. female organ of copulation
9. — — — T — —   9. pouch that covers the testes
10. — — — — — I — —   10. infertility
11. — — O — — — —   11. sexually transmitted disease
12. — — — N — — — —   12. inflammation of the vagina

Anatomy Review. *Male Tract.* Using colored pencils or crayons, color the organs of the male reproductive tract as indicated. Trace the pathway of sperm. Follow from origin to leaving the body and color the structures red.

13. urinary bladder—yellow

14. penis—blue

15. testis—brown

16. prostate gland—green

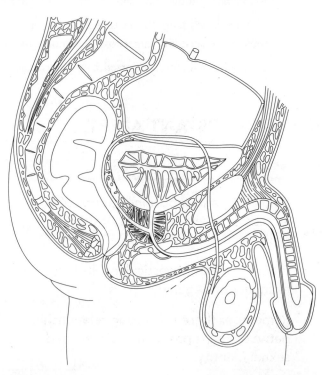

Female Tract. Using colored pencils or crayons, color the organs of the female tract as indicated. Then in red trace the pathway of an egg from point of origin to uterus.

17. uterine walls—yellow

18. right ovary—blue

19. right oviduct—green

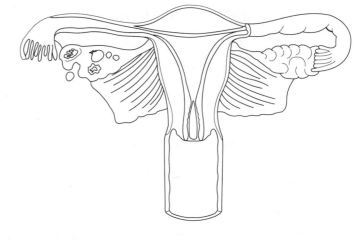

20. labia majora—red

21. clitoris—yellow

22. urinary meatus—green

23. labia minora—blue

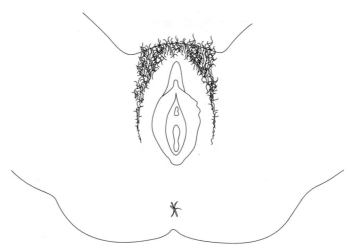

Completion.   Complete the statements in the spaces provided.

24. A common enlargement of the prostate gland is due to benign _____ .

25. The tube-like organ passing through the center of the prostate gland is the _____ .

26. A major problem for men suffering from the condition named in statement 24 is urinary _____
_____ .

27. Men undergoing prostatectomy are apt to be _____
upset by the thought of the procedure.

28. The patient returning from prostate surgery will have a _____ in place.

29. Testicular self-examination should be performed at least once each _____ .

30. The best time to perform testicular self-examination is during a _____ .

31. A colporrhaphy is performed to tighten the _____ walls.

32. An uncomfortable and distressing problem associated with a cystocele is urinary _____
_____ .

33. Vulvovaginitis that is often caused by *Candida albicans* is a _____ infection.

34. A simple test used to detect possible cancer of the cervix is the _____ .

35. A _____ is a surgical procedure employed to help diagnose conditions of the uterus.

36. Removal of the fallopian tubes is known as a bilateral _____.

37. Following a mastectomy, bed linen should be checked, because blood may drain to the _____ _____ of the dressing.

38. Vaginitis caused by *Trichomonas vaginalis* is associated with a foul-smelling discharge called _____ _____ .

39. In early stages, females infected with *Neisseria gonorrhea* are frequently _____ that they have been infected.

40. The organism causing syphilis is known to pass from mother to child through the _____ _____ .

41. *Chlamydia* infections can cause serious _____.

42. Cancer of the testes may require removal by a surgical procedure called an _____.

Brief Answers Briefly answer the following questions.

43. What three functions do the male and female reproductive tracts have in common?

    a. _____

    b. _____

    c. _____

44. What are three surgical procedures used to perform a prostatectomy and how do they differ?

    Technique (approach)   **Difference**

    a. _____

    _____

    b. _____

    _____

    c. _____

    _____

45. What special care should you give postoperatively when caring for the prostatectomy patient?

    a. _____

    b. _____

    c. _____

    d. _____

    e. _____

    f. _____

46. What nursing care procedures might be ordered following an anterior colporrhaphy?

    a. _____

    b. _____

    c. _____

    d. _____

47. Why is there an attempt to leave at least part of an ovary when a hysterectomy is needed in a younger woman?

_____

48. What special postoperative care is required for a patient following a panhysterectomy?

a. _____

b. _____

c. _____

d. _____

e. _____

f. _____

49. When and how should a woman check her breasts?

a. _____

b. _____

c. _____

d. _____

e. _____

f. _____

50. What are the names and causative organisms of six sexually transmitted diseases described in your text?

	Disease	Organism
a.		
b.		
c.		
d.		
e.		
f.		

51. How should the procedure for testicular self-examination be performed?

a. _____

b. _____

c. _____

d. _____

52. What are two problems associated with rectoceles?

a. _____

b. _____

53. Why is it important to maintain good circulation in the patient who has just experienced a panhysterectomy?

_____

54. What are six signs or symptoms of a breast tumor?

a. _____

b. _____

c. _____

d. _____

e. _____

f. _____

Clinical Situations. Briefly describe how a nursing assistant should react to the following situations.

55. A patient expresses concern about being able to perform sexually after a prostatectomy.

_____

56. A patient is to have a lumpectomy and wants to know if the entire breast will be removed.

_____

_____

57. Your patient is scheduled for a suprapubic prostatectomy. He expresses to you his concerns about the possibility of being impotent following surgery.

_____

RELATING TO THE NURSING PROCESS

Write the step of the nursing process that is related to the nursing assistant action.

Nursing Assistant Action	Nursing Process Step
58. The nursing assistant reports to the nurse that the patient is complaining of itching and has a watery vaginal discharge.	_____
59. The nursing assistant checks the bed to the back for bleeding following a mastectomy.	_____
60. The nursing assistant informs the nurse of the grief and frustrations the postoperative mastectomy patient is expressing.	_____
61. The nursing assistant inserts the douche nozzle slowly, while the fluid is flowing, in an upward and backward motion.	_____
62. The nursing assistant carefully notes and reports color and amount of drainage from all areas for the patient who has had a prostatectomy.	_____

DEVELOPING GREATER INSIGHT

63. Think about how you would feel if you found a lump in your breast or testes. What if it turned out to be malignant?

64. Discuss reasons why people tend to be particularly sensitive when there is disease or injury involving the reproductive organs.

65. Think about why it is important to use standard precautions when caring for patients with sexually transmitted diseases.

UNIT 44   Rehabilitation and Restorative Services

OBJECTIVES

As a result of this unit, you will be able to:

■ Spell and define terms.

■ Describe the differences between rehabilitation and restorative care.

■ List five members of the interdisciplinary team.

■ Describe the role of the nursing assistant in rehabilitation.

■ Describe the principles of rehabilitation.

■ List the elements of successful rehabilitation/restorative care.

■ List six complications resulting from inactivity.

■ Describe four perceptual deficits.

■ Describe four approaches used for restorative programs.

■ Describe the guidelines for implementing restorative programs.

UNIT SUMMARY

Rehabilitation and restorative care are designed to help patients reach an optimal level of personal ability. The most successful programs:

■ Begin as soon as possible

■ Stress abilities

■ Treat the whole patient

Care is planned by an interdisciplinary health care team, of which the nursing assistant is an important member. Nursing assistants participate in the restorative program by:

■ Knowing and following the stated nursing health care plan.

■ Supporting the patient's efforts toward independence.

■ Assisting the nurses with procedures designed to meet specific patient needs.

■ Maintaining the patient's nutrition.

Nursing assistants can make a valuable contribution to the success of the patient's program by demonstrating a consistent, positive, and patient attitude.

NURSING ASSISTANT ALERT

Action	Benefit
Give patient opportunities to make decisions whenever possible.	Adds to patient's sense of control

Action	Benefit
Treat patient with dignity at all times.	Encourages patient's self-esteem and fosters attitude of cooperation.
Be encouraging and give praise.	Promotes positive attitude in patient and inspires him or her to keep trying.
Know the care plan and follow it.	Assures that restorative/rehabilitation program will be focused and consistent.

ACTIVITIES

Vocabulary Exercise. Using the definitions, write the proper words in the spaces provided.

1. A disability that prevents a person from fulfilling a role that is normal for that person. _____

2. Physician who specializes in rehabilitation. _____

3. Ordinary items that are modified for a specific patient. _____

4. Process that assists the patient to reach an optimal level of ability. _____

5. Impairment that affects the person's ability to perform an activity that a person of that age would usually be able to do. _____

Completion. Complete the following statements in the spaces provided. Select the proper terms from the list provided.

care	disability	disease or injury	handicap
influence	optimum level of performance	problems	rehabilitation
retraining	same approach	self-care deficit	strength

6. Rehabilitation refers to a process in which the patient strives for the _____.

7. A person with paralysis suffers from a _____.

8. A person who has been in bed for a long time because of heart disease may require _____.

9. All the different disciplines that take part in rehabilitation work together to resolve _____ and plan _____.

10. Any activity a patient is capable of doing is considered a _____.

11. Patients and family _____ the emotional and mental health of patients who are being rehabilitated.

12. A patient who cannot complete any or all of the ADLs independently is said to have a _____.

13. Damage to the brain usually occurs because of _____.

14. Restorative programs are sometimes referred to as _____ programs.

15. It is important that everyone working with a patient in restorative care use the _____.

Brief Answers. Briefly answer the following questions.

16. List five goals that rehabilitation and restorative activities share.

a. _____

b. _____

c. _____

d. _____

e. _____

17. State seven activities that are included in the tasks of daily living (ADL).

a. _____ e. _____

b. _____ f. _____

c. _____ g. _____

d. _____

18. List three goals the interdisciplinary team has for a person with a handicap.

a. _____

b. _____

c. _____

19. Name five professionals, other than nurses and physicians, who are involved in the rehabilitative process.

a. _____

b. _____

c. _____

d. _____

e. _____

20. List six rehabilitation activities in which the nursing assistant will assist.

a. _____

b. _____

c. _____

d. _____

e. _____

f. _____

21. Write the four principles that form the foundation for successful rehabilitation or restorative care.

a. _____

b. _____

c. _____

d. _____

22. State six examples of conditions that limit a person's ability to do self-care.

a. _____ d. _____

b. _____ e. _____

c. _____ f. _____

23. List six examples of perceptual deficits.

    a. _____

    b. _____

    c. _____

    d. _____

    e. _____

    f. _____

24. Name four approaches used in restorative programs.

    a. _____

    b. _____

    c. _____

    d. _____

25. Describe the type of environment that benefits patients as they attempt to succeed in a restorative program.

    _____

    _____

Clinical Situations. Briefly describe how a nursing assistant should react to the following situations.

26. Mr. Fronzoni is very frustrated as the nursing assistant explains how to put his socks on before the shoes. _____

    _____

27. Mr. Tracy has a roommate who repeatedly interrupts as the nursing assistant tries to help Mr. Tracy hold his glass. _____

    _____

28. Mrs. Davis is frustrated this morning and says that her progress is "just too slow." _____

    _____

29. The nursing assistant is assigned for the first time this morning to care for Mrs. Washington, who needs help with her self-feeding program. _____

    _____

30. Mr. Smythe is left-handed and has an adaptive device for his left hand, which is on his bedside table as he attempts to brush his teeth. _____

    _____

31. Mrs. Missel is unable to gather the necessary equipment to give herself a bath and then carry out the procedure.

    _____

32. Mrs. Wexford has difficulty manipulating her clothing when she uses the toilet. She is able to stand and sit independently. _____

    _____

33. Mr. Surgernt can hold his toothbrush and put it in his mouth, but then just holds it there. _____

    _____

34. Mrs. Malone is in a restorative program in the skilled care facility, but seems bored and restless between activity sessions. _____

    _____

35. Complete the chart by placing an x in the appropriate space.

   Mr. Cochran is admitted for rehabilitation. Mr. Ward is admitted to the same skilled care facility, but his goal is restoration. How does rehabilitation differ from restoration?

Activity	Rehabilitation	Restoration
a. OBRA requires that care *must* be carried out in a skilled care facility.		
b. Goal is to increase the patient's quality of life.		
c. May be provided in a general acute care hospital.		
d. Usually more aggressive and intense.		
e. Slower therapies over weeks, months, or indefinitely.		
f. Requires the skills of many different therapists.		
g. Primarily a nursing responsibility with consultation.		

RELATING TO THE NURSING PROCESS

Write the step of the nursing process that is related to the nursing assistant action.

Nursing Assistant Action	Nursing Process Step
36. The nursing assistant begins passive exercises and positioning for Mrs. Burton, who is stable after a right-sided brain attack.	
37. The nursing assistant encourages Mr. Jackson, who has poor strength in his dominant right hand, as he tries to feed himself with his left hand.	
38. The nursing assistant participates in team care conferences.	
39. The nursing assistant reports that Mrs. Parson is able to move her hands but is unable to select and hold items.	

DEVELOPING GREATER INSIGHT

40. With a classmate acting as a nursing assistant, practice trying to use your nondominant hand to eat, secure your shoes, and put on your clothes. Discuss how it makes you feel.

41. When first waking in the morning, lie in bed and think how frustrating it would be not to be able to carry out your morning hygiene routine.

42. Borrow a wheelchair and try to navigate around your community or school campus. Discuss the problems you encounter when you can't use your legs to walk.

UNIT 45   Obstetrical Patient and Neonate

OBJECTIVES

As a result of this unit, you will be able to:
- Spell and define terms.
- Assist in the prenatal care of the normal pregnant woman.
- List reportable observations of patients in the prenatal period.
- Assist in care of the normal postpartum patient.
- Properly change a perineal pad.
- Recognize reportable observations of patients in the postpartum period.
- Recognize reportable signs and symptoms of urine retention in the postpartum period.
- Assist in care of the normal newborn.
- Demonstrate three methods of safely holding a baby.
- Assist in carrying out the discharge procedures for mother and infant.

UNIT SUMMARY

The care of the obstetrical patient is a very specialized area of medicine. It includes:
- Supervision of the health of the mother throughout the prenatal, labor and delivery, and postpartum periods to discharge.
- Care of the neonate.

    The nursing assistant may participate in this care under the close direction of the professional staff if facility policy permits.
    A thorough understanding of your responsibilities and close attention to the details of care help ensure a successful and safe pregnancy and delivery.
    All the procedures presented in this unit require advanced training and supervision before you attempt to perform them. In addition, you may do so only under proper authorization.

NURSING ASSISTANT ALERT

Action	Benefit
Follow orders carefully during the prenatal, delivery, and postpartum periods.	Helps ensure a successful and safe pregnancy and delivery.
Keep one hand near the baby when weighing it.	Prevents injury of the infant.
Handle and carry babies securely in an approved manner.	Protects the baby from injury.

Action	Benefit
Be open and supportive of parents faced with difficult or unsuccessful pregnancies and deliveries.	Provides essential emotional support when parents need it the most.

ACTIVITIES

Vocabulary Exercise. Each line has four different spellings of a word. Circle the correctly spelled word.

1. lokia	lochia	logia	lochea
2. neonat	nionat	nionate	neonate
3. fetal	fetie	fietal	fetyl
4. epescotomy	episiotomy	epysiotomy	episiotomie
5. umbalical	umbilicale	umbilical	umbelical
6. placenta	placentar	placenter	plecentar
7. effase	affase	afface	efface
8. amneotic	amniotic	amiotic	ammiotic

Definitions. Define the following terms.

9. amniocentesis _____

10. lochia _____

11. postpartum _____

12. lactation _____

13. episiotomy _____

14. neonate _____

15. fundus _____

16. placenta _____

17. dilation _____

18. amniotic fluid _____

Completion. Complete the following statements in the spaces provided.

19. A clinic that provides care during and following pregnancy is called an _____ clinic.

20. The first trimester includes months _____ of the pregnancy.

21. Early signs of pregnancy include _____.

22. The fetus in the uterus receives nourishment through the _____.

23. The afterbirth is called the _____.

24. Parental interaction with the baby is believed to encourage _____.

25. The technique to detect possible abnormalities which permits direct visualization of the fetus is called

_____.

26. The dilation stage of labor begins with the first regular _____ and ends when the _____ is fully dilated.

27. During the period of dilation, the cervix opens up and _____ out.

28. An instrument used to check the well-being of the baby during labor is called a _____ .

29. Both mother and child must be _____ before either is moved from the delivery room.

30. If a fetus is in distress, it may be necessary to perform a _____ delivery.

31. The usual part of the baby to be delivered first is the _____.

32. A soft and enlarging postpartum uterus must be reported because it indicates excessive _____.

33. While weighing a baby, never turn your _____ to the scale and keep one _____ over the baby at all times.

34. If it is necessary to carry the infant in your arms, always _____ through a doorway.

35. Be sure to wash hands _____ and _____ handling each child and after each _____ change.

36. A circumcision should be checked _____.

37. PKU is detected by a _____ test.

38. The baby is dressed in _____ clothes for discharge.

39. A technique that can be used to help firm up a soft uterus is to _____ the fundus.

40. A new mother should be encouraged to void within the first _____ hours postpartum.

41. Inability to void following delivery should be reported because a full bladder can cause postpartum _____.

42. The "cramping" mothers feel postpartum is due to the uterus _____.

43. A swelling just above the pubis and complaints of urgency but with voiding of less than 200 mL indicates _____.

44. When removing a soiled perineal pad, always wear _____, fold the soiled side of the pad _____, and wrap the pad in a _____.

45. Never dispose of soiled perineal pads in the _____.

46. Mothers who are breast-feeding should be instructed to wash their breasts using a _____ motion from _____ outward.

47. The Apgar scoring is an evaluation of the _____ which is made at _____ minute and _____ minutes after birth.

48. An Apgar score of 9 indicates the neonate is in _____ condition.

49. The baby must be kept warm until his _____ stabilizes.

50. In the nursery, the _____, weight, and vital signs are measured.

51. A pregnancy should test positive within _____ days after conception.

Brief Answers. Briefly answer the following questions.

52. What is meant when we say the length of pregnancy is divided into three trimesters?

_____

_____

53. Which care is given to the mother during the prenatal period?

a. _____

b. _____

c. _____

d. _____

54. What observations during the prenatal visit must be reported to the nurse or physician?

   a. _____

   b. _____

   c. _____

   d. _____

55. What are three anesthetic approaches frequently used for a vaginal delivery?

   a. _____

   b. _____

   c. _____

56. List three benefits of natural childbirth.

   a. _____

   b. _____

   c. _____

57. Identify three techniques used to examine the fetus in the uterus.

   a. _____

   b. _____

   c. _____

58. Besides routine anesthesia, what four special care procedures should be carried out for the patient who has had a cesarean section?

   a. _____

   b. _____

   c. _____

   d. _____

59. What three techniques might be ordered to relieve the perineal discomfort of an episiotomy?

   a. _____

   b. _____

   c. _____

60. What are two values of colostrum to the baby?

   a. _____

   b. _____

61. What five areas are evaluated during Apgar scoring?

   a. _____

   b. _____

   c. _____

   d. _____

   e. _____

62. List ways of caring for the breast of the nursing mother.

    a. _____

    b. _____

    c. _____

    d. _____

    e. _____

63. How should the baby be lifted from the crib?

    a. _____

    b. _____

Clinical Situations. Briefly explain how the nursing assistant should react to the following situations.

64. The new mother is very uncomfortable when she tries to sit. _____

_____

_____

65. The young mother is told the form of care in this hospital is "rooming in" and asks what this means. _____

_____

_____

66. The new mother has returned to your care in the postpartum area.

    a. _____

    b. _____

    c. _____

    d. _____

    e. _____

Identification.

67. Write the names of the parts or structures indicated in the spaces provided.

    a. _____

    b. _____

    c. _____

    d. _____

    e. _____

    f. _____

    g. _____

    h. _____

RELATING TO THE NURSING PROCESS

Write the step of the nursing process that is related to the nursing assistant action.

Nursing Assistant Action	Nursing Process Step
68. Working in a prenatal clinic, the nursing assistant weighs patients and measures blood pressure.	_____
69. The nursing assistant helps other staff members transfer the newly delivered mother from stretcher to bed.	_____
70. The nursing assistant checks the vital signs as ordered following a cesarean section.	_____
71. The nursing assistant measures and records the first postpartum voiding.	_____
72. The nursing assistant immediately reports to the nurse when she finds the uterus of the new postpartum patient becoming soft and enlarged.	_____

DEVELOPING GREATER INSIGHT

73. Identify what special help a new mother may require because she doesn't remain in the hospital very long for care.

74. Discuss with classmates the information you or your partner would need to know when you learn you or she is pregnant.

75. Visit a prenatal clinic. Report back to the class on your observations.

UNIT 46   Pediatric Patient

OBJECTIVES

As a result of this unit, you will be able to:

- Spell and define terms.

- Describe the major developmental tasks for each pediatric age group.

- Describe how to foster growth and development for hospitalized pediatric patients.

- Describe how to maintain a safe environment for the pediatric patient.

- Discuss the role of parents and siblings of the hospitalized pediatric patient.

- Demonstrate the following procedures:

    Procedure 119 Admitting a Pediatric Patient
    Procedure 120 Weighing the Pediatric Patient
    Procedure 121 Changing Crib Linens
    Procedure 122 Changing Crib Linens (Infant in Crib)
    Procedure 123 Measuring Temperature
    Procedure 124 Determining Heart Rate (Pulse)
    Procedure 125 Counting Respiratory Rate
    Procedure 126 Measuring Blood Pressure
    Procedure 127 Bottle-Feeding the Infant
    Procedure 128 Burping (Method A)
    Procedure 129 Burping (Method B)

UNIT SUMMARY

This unit provides the nursing assistant with information on giving safe care to the hospitalized pediatric patient. Because children differ in age, size, and developmental level, five developmental levels are described:

- Infancy

- Toddler

- Preschooler

- School-age

- Adolescent

For each age group, suggestions are offered to promote normal growth and development while maintaining a safe environment for the hospitalized pediatric patient.

Families are important to the pediatric patient. Because the family can also be affected by the child's hospitalization, suggestions are provided to promote and encourage a family-centered approach to care.

NURSING ASSISTANT ALERT

Action	Benefit
Maintain a safe environment.	Keeps child safe from injury.
Provide opportunity for decision making.	Supports the child's need for growing independence.
Familiarize yourself with the usual changes that occur at different chronological ages. Recognize that people reach developmental stages at different rates.	Helps to ensure individualization of patient care.

ACTIVITIES

Vocabulary Exercise. Put a circle around the word defined.

1. fantasies

2. to promote

3. brothers and sisters

4. to move backward

5. a child from birth to 1 year

6. to move away from center

7. children from 6 to 12 years

8. children from 13 to 18 years

9. pertaining to children

```
P Q S A O K F F D I E J K E G L
H A U F T D O H K I N F A N T T
E D E V I A T E G O P F I L E D
P O M B C F O T C K I K S E D L
G L O D L R D F T O N L R E P S
S E B F O S I B L I N G S H L T
L S A C F L I O H J E A D I F M
E C L N F O S T E R J I W R B N
S E L C K Y L G I E K A N H U S
X N J F T A K E I L G E P P E G
G T K S C H O O L A G E E R G K
L E O I X F J I L H S N D W I T
R E G R E S S B O U O F I E K M
H A J C K I F W C A V S A A E E
M P A D I B A I L O M B T H Y T
R G H B O D F I D H G K R E A B
B E R T H B N R Y O I K I L D G
L X C J L E R D Q A S E C C I G
```

Completion. Complete the statements in the spaces provided.

10. What are two ways pediatric departments are usually organized?

a. _____

b. _____

11. Who provides the medical and social history when the patient is a child?

_____

12. What information about the pediatric patient might you learn from the history form that will help you in the care you will give?

a. _____

b. _____

c. _____

13. Why is "rooming in" with a pediatric patient a good idea?

_____

14. How will the infant change in the first year of life?

a. _____

b. _____

15. What is meant by the infant's "developmental milestones"?

_____

_____

16. What is the primary psychosocial development task for the infant?

_____

17. How might you foster the achievement of the infant's developmental task?

_____

_____

18. At what age does the infant usually begin to display a fear of strangers?

_____

19. What are three appropriate toys for the infant?

a. _____

b. _____

c. _____

20. How should the care of an infant be organized?

_____

_____

21. If a toddler is unable to stand on an upright scale, how may he be weighed?

_____

_____

22. What factors would increase the infant's heart rate and respirations?

a. _____

b. _____

c. _____

23. When should the other vital signs be measured when a rectal temperature is to be measured? _____

24. How might an infant's sucking needs be met when she cannot eat?

_____

25. If the toddler is toilet trained, what information would be helpful for you to know?

_____

_____

26. What is a major fear of the preschooler? _____

_____

27. Because preschoolers have a limited concept of time, how should you explain when something will occur? _____

_____

28. How could you foster the need the school-age child has for accomplishment? _____

_____

29. How may an adolescent view the nursing assistant and other caregivers? _____

_____

30. Who are the most important people to the adolescent? _____

_____

31. Altered appearance upsets teenagers' feelings about their _____ .

Brief Answers. Briefly answer the following questions.

32. List seven safety measures related to the infant.

a. _____

b. _____

c. _____

d. _____

e. _____

f. _____

g. _____

33. What actions might you take to reassure a toddler when "rooming in" is not possible?

a. _____

b. _____

c. _____

d. _____

34. What are five activities you might choose for a toddler?

a. _____

b. _____

c. _____

d. _____

e. _____

35. What are nine safety guidelines when caring for a toddler?

a. _____

b. _____

c. _____

d. _____

e. _____

f. _____

g. _____

h. _____

i. _____

36. What are three ways the school-age children might demonstrate his need for help without asking?

    a. _____

    b. _____

    c. _____

37. What are three things you should do to make a hospital stay less difficult for the adolescent?

    a. _____

    b. _____

    c. _____

Clinical Situations. Briefly describe how a nursing assistant should react to the following situations.

38. The toddler who is weaned cries for a bottle. _____

    _____

39. The toddler is having a temper tantrum. _____

    _____

40. The teenager doesn't want to go to sleep after the television has been shut off.

    _____

    _____

RELATING TO THE NURSING PROCESS

Write the step of the nursing process that is related to the nursing assistant action.

Nursing Assistant Action	Nursing Process Step
41. The nursing assistant measures and weighs the child on admission to the pediatric unit.	_____
42. The nursing assistant helps stabilize the preschooler's arm while offering comforting support during blood withdrawal.	_____
43. The nursing assistant finds ways to occupy a roommate when a school-age patient is visited by a tutor.	_____
44. The nursing assistant always keep the crib sides up when the toddler is in the crib.	_____
45. The nursing assistant discusses with the nurse activities for the recuperating toddler in her care.	_____

DEVELOPING GREATER INSIGHT

46. Describe as many different types of "family units" as you can.

47. Discuss reasons why teens join gangs. How will you feel about caring for a teen injured in a gang fight?

UNIT 47   Special Advanced Procedures

OBJECTIVES

As a result of this unit—and with advanced training—you will be able to:

■ Spell and define terms.

■ Demonstrate the following procedures:

Procedure 130 Testing for Occult Blood Using Hemoccult® and Developer
Procedure 131 Testing for Occult Blood Using Hematest® Reagent Tablets
Procedure 132 Collecting a Urine Specimen Through a Drainage Port
Procedure 133 Giving Routine Stoma Care (Colostomy)
Procedure 134 Routine Care of an Ileostomy (with Patient in Bed)

UNIT SUMMARY

As a nursing assistant you should be willing to learn and grow in your chosen field, always bearing in mind your ethical and legal limitations.

■ Material in this unit introduces techniques that may be assigned to the experienced nursing assistant who has received advanced training and who has demonstrated skill and proficiency.

■ These procedures must be carried out under proper supervision and authorization, because any errors might result in a greater likelihood of injury to the patient or inaccuracy of test results.

NURSING ASSISTANT ALERT

Action	Benefit
Carry out only those procedures that are within the guidelines for nursing assistant responsibilities.	Legally protects both patient and caregiver.
Be sure to have proper authorization and supervision before acting.	Ensures care will be safely and properly given.
Be willing to learn, guided by ethical and legal limitations.	Contributes to a growth environment in which the caregiver's skills can be upgraded.

ACTIVITIES

Vocabulary Exercise. Unscramble the words introduced in this unit and define them.

1. LIAPPACNE   _____

2. OSEMLITOY   _____

3. TMSOOY   _____

4. OPTR   _____

5. OTSAM   _____

6. TSYOMOCLO   _____

Completion. Complete the statements in the spaces provided.

7. When using a HemaCombistix® strip, do not touch the test areas of the strip with the _____.

8. Fecal samples should be taken from different parts of the _____ when using Hemoccult® and
developer.

9. Presence of blood when tested by Hemoccult® and developer is indicated by a _____ of the smear.

10. Some closed urinary systems have a _____ for the collection of a urine sample.

11. Clamp the catheter _____ before collecting a urine sample from a closed drainage system.

12. If there is no port in a closed drainage system, the area where the catheter joins the drainage tube must be cleansed with _____ before disconnection.

13. The initial irrigations of a colostomy will be performed by the _____.

14. The drainage from a ileostomy is in a _____ form and contains _____ enzymes.

15. The drainage from an ileostomy is very _____ , so careful stoma care is essential.

16. A Karaya gum ring can be loosened from the skin around the stoma by using a few drops of
_____.

17. Each facility has established policies that are consistent with _____ regulations.

18. Some advanced procedures considered routine for some caregivers would _____ appropriate for others.

19. When performing tests for occult blood, always _____.

20. Stool samples should be obtained using a _____.

Brief Answers. Briefly answer the following questions.

21. For what is the HemaCombistix® used to test? _____

22. What equipment would you need to test for occult blood in feces using Hemoccult® and developer?

a. _____

b. _____

c. _____

d. _____

23. What equipment will be needed to collect a urine specimen through the drainage port of a closed system?

    a. _____

    b. _____

    c. _____

    d. _____

    e. _____

    f. _____

    g. _____

    h. _____

    i. _____

24. How might you assist the colostomy patient to keep the stoma comfortable?

    a. _____

    b. _____

    c. _____

25. What factors influence the scope and types of assignments given to nursing assistants?

    a. _____

    b. _____

    c. _____

    d. _____

26. What factors must be kept in mind when you are assigned to collect urine from a patient on a closed urinary drainage system?

    a. _____

    b. _____

    c. _____

27. Why must a fresh urine sample not be taken from the bag when the patient is on closed urinary drainage?

    _____

28. How is the port in a closed drainage system disinfected before inserting the needle to withdraw a sample? _____

    _____

29. What are three problems associated with a colostomy stoma?

    a. _____

    b. _____

    c. _____

30. What factor determines the nature of the feces eliminated through a colostomy? _____

    _____

Clinical Situations. Briefly describe how a nursing assistant should react to the following situations.

31. The patient has a small amount of mushy stool around her stoma when you remove the stoma bag. _____

    _____

32. A barrier cream has been applied around the patient's colostomy stoma, but the seal is not secure. _____

    _____

33. It is necessary to remove the adhesive wafer around the stoma. How can you be sure to select a new wafer of the proper size?

_____

34. You are giving stoma care to a patient with an ileostomy. What are your primary responsibilities? _____

_____

_____

RELATING TO THE NURSING PROCESS

Write the step of the nursing process that is related to the nursing assistant action.

Nursing Assistant Action   **Nursing Process Step**

35. The nursing assistant wears disposable gloves when cleaning around a colostomy stoma.

_____

36. The nursing assistant shows the nurse the results after performing the test for occult blood using Hemoccult® and developer.

_____

37. The nursing assistant reports that there was a small amount of liquid stool in the disposable colostomy drainage pouch.

_____

DEVELOPING GREATER INSIGHT

38. At home draw a circle on your abdomen with lipstick or marker. Now look in the mirror and try to imagine that you must use that opening to eliminate solid wastes.

39. Discuss reasons why it is so important to keep the area around a colostomy stoma dry. Explain why it is more difficult to keep the area around an ileostomy stoma dry.

UNIT 48 Response to Basic Emergencies

OBJECTIVES

As a result of this unit, you will be able to:

- Spell and define terms.

- Recognize emergency situations that require urgent care.

- Be able to evaluate situations and determine the sequence of appropriate actions to be taken.

- Recognize the need for CPR.

- Identify the signs, symptoms, and treatment of common emergency situations such as:

    Fainting
    Heart attack
    Bleeding
    Shock
    Brain attack (stroke)
    Thermal injuries
    Poisoning
    Choking
    Cardiac arrest
    Seizure
- Demonstrate the following procedures:

    Procedure 135 Adult CPR, One Rescuer
    Procedure 136 Adult CPR, Two-Person
    Procedure 137 Heimlich Maneuver—Abdominal Thrusts
    Procedure 138 Assisting the Adult Who Has an Obstructed Airway and Becomes Unconscious
    Procedure 139 CPR for Infants
    Procedure 140 Obstructed Airway: Conscious Infant
    Procedure 141 Obstructed Airway: Unconscious Infant
    Procedure 142 CPR for Children, One Rescuer
    Procedure 143 Child with Foreign Body Airway Obstruction

UNIT SUMMARY

Emergency situations can occur without warning at any time. A person who has been specially trained in the techniques of first aid can be of great service.

- Remain calm.

- Never overestimate your abilities.

- Use the special skills you have been taught wisely.

Special training will enable you to assess injuries and know the proper steps to follow in:

- Calling for help.

- Carrying out lifesaving skills such as CPR.
- Controlling bleeding.
- Helping victims of disease and trauma.

NURSING ASSISTANT ALERT

Action	Benefit
Never overestimate your abilities.	Prevents injuries due to improper actions.
Follow only approved actions.	Can be lifesaving. Avoids legal liability.

ACTIVITIES

Vocabulary Exercise. Complete the puzzle by filling in the missing letters of words found in this unit. Use the definitions to help you discover these words.

1.	——— U——	1.	injury
2.	—— R———	2.	stoppage of heartbeat
3.	G	3.	
4.	————— E——	4.	an unintended occurrence
5.	—————— N——	5.	a situation that develops rapidly and unexpectedly
6.	———— T———————	6.	emergency cardiac condition
		7.	disturbance of oxygen supply to the tissues and return of blood to heart
7.	——— C—		
8.	———— A——	8.	to raise
9	—— R	9.	cardiopulmonary resuscitation
10.	— E———————	10.	loss of blood

Completion. Complete the statements in the spaces provided.

11. Your actions should never place the victim in additional _____.

12. First aid techniques are taught as a specific course by the _____.

13. Certification in CPR is provided in courses by the _____ and the American Red Cross.

14. In an emergency situation, always refer to someone who has greater _____ or _____.

15. When you provide first aid, you must deal with the victim's _____ as well as the victim's physical injuries.

16. The first step when arriving at the scene of an accident is to _____ the situation.

17. If you are in a medical facility when an accident occurs, you should _____ for help and keep the patient _____.

18. The national number for emergency help is _____.

19. The most common cause of airway obstruction is _____, so pulling the _____ forward often opens the airway.

20. If oxygen is denied to the body, the most sensitive organ, the _____, may suffer permanent damage.

21. Checking for breathing should take _____.

22. Care that must be given immediately to prevent loss of life is called _____.

23. When moving a victim, always move him as a single _____.

24. The Heimlich maneuver refers to the technique of performing _____ thrusts.

25. If finger sweeps are needed, the finger should not poke _____ because it may push the object down.

26. A disturbance of the oxygen supply to the tissues and return of blood to the heart is defined as _____.

27. The victim in shock should be kept _____ down with feet elevated.

28. The loss of heart function is called _____.

29. Seizures do not always follow the same _____.

30. In a grand mal seizure, the patient must be protected against _____ himself.

31. Following a grand mal seizure, the patient may be _____ and _____ for a time and feel very tired.

32. A good way to move a victim of electric shock away from the source of electricity is to use something made of _____.

Brief Answers. Briefly answer the following questions.

33. What four basic actions should be taken in all emergency situations?

    a. _____

    b. _____

    c. _____

    d. _____

34. What facts should be included when calling the emergency number?

    a. _____

    b. _____

    c. _____

    d. _____

    e. _____

35. What two types of care are included in first aid?

    a. _____

    b. _____

36. What are six life-threatening situations that require immediate first aid treatment?

    a. _____

    b. _____

    c. _____

    d. _____

    e. _____

    f. _____

37. What are four ways to summon help for an accident victim in a health facility?

    a. _____

    b. _____

    c. _____

    d. _____

38. How should you check for breathing activity?

    a. _____

    b. _____

39. What order of victim's responses should be checked when providing urgent care?

    a. _____

    b. _____

    c. _____

    d. _____

    e. _____

40. How would you describe the distress signals of choking? _____

    _____

    _____

41. What steps should you follow to prevent additional blood loss in a bleeding victim?

    a. _____

    b. _____

    c. _____

    d. _____

    e. _____

    f. _____

42. What are the early signs of shock?

    a. _____

    b. _____

    c. _____

    d. _____

    e. _____

43. What signs and symptoms might indicate the victim is having a heart attack?

    a. _____

    b. _____

    c. _____

    d. _____

    e. _____

Clinical Situations. Briefly describe how a nursing assistant should react to the following situations.

44. You are the first person on the scene of an auto accident. One person has been thrown out of the car and is lying beside the car, which is on fire. Describe your first action.

   _____

45. You discover the husband of your home client on the floor of the basement near a frayed electrical wire. What is your first action? _____

   _____

46. You are in a dining area and an ambulatory patient grasps his throat, makes high-pitched sounds, and is unable to speak. _____

   _____

   _____

   _____

RELATING TO THE NURSING PROCESS

Write the step of the nursing process that is related to the nursing assistant action.

Nursing Assistant Action	Nursing Process Step
47. The nursing assistant, finding a patient on the floor, first checks for consciousness.	_____
48. The nursing assistant finds an unconscious patient and signals immediately for help.	_____
49. The patient stumbles, injuring her knee, which begins to bleed. The nursing assistant applies direct pressure with his gloved hand.	_____
50. The nursing assistant encourages the patient to rest quietly after a seizure.	_____
51. After summoning help for the heart attack victim, the nursing assistant remains with the patient to offer emotional support.	_____

UNIT 49   Employment Opportunities and Career Growth

OBJECTIVES

As a result of this unit, you will be able to:

- Spell and define terms.
- List nine objectives to be met in obtaining and maintaining employment.
- Follow a process for self-appraisal.
- Name sources of employment for nursing assistants.
- Prepare a résumé and a letter of resignation.
- List steps for a successful interview.
- List the requirements that must be met when accepting employment.
- List steps for continuing development in your career.

UNIT SUMMARY

Finding the right employment after completion of your nursing assistant program can be easier if you set objectives and meet each one in a systematic fashion.

The steps to take include:

- Appraising your assets and limitations.
- Searching the job market.
- Securing and holding the position.
- Properly resigning when it is time to make a career change.

Learning is a lifelong process. It may involve additional education and the ability to leave one position to move to another.

NURSING ASSISTANT ALERT

Action	Benefit
Be honest in your self-appraisals.	Provides accurate assessments upon which decisions can be appropriately made.
Conduct yourself in an ethical and proper manner.	Assures success in developing and maintaining successful employment opportunities.
Recognize that learning is a lifetime task.	Keeps your knowledge and skills updated.

ACTIVITIES

Vocabulary Exercise. Write the words forming the circle and define them.

1. _____

2. _____

3. _____

4. _____

Completion. Complete the following statements in the spaces provided.

5. One of the first steps in self-appraisal is to list all your _____ and _____.

6. It is important to think through possible _____ to any limitations to employment.

7. Preference for caring for a particular type of patient could influence your _____ options.

8. Home _____ and transportation are factors that might limit employment.

9. Talking with friends and colleagues about opportunities is called _____.

10. A written summary of work history is called a _____.

11. Always obtain _____ before giving a name as a reference.

12. References should know you well, but not be _____.

13. Clothing should be _____ and _____ for an interview.

14. It is important to be on _____ for an interview.

15. In a new work situation, there is much to learn from the examples of _____ staff workers.

16. When it is necessary to resign, do so in a _____ manner.

Brief Answers Briefly answer the following questions.

17. What will you specifically look for when seeking employment through the classified ads?

   a. _____

   b. _____

   c. _____

   d. _____

18. What information should not be included in a résumé?

   a. _____

   b. _____

   c. _____

   d. _____

   e. _____

Practical Applications. Briefly describe the actions the nursing assistant might take in the following situations.

19. A classmate asks where nursing assistants might be employed.

_____

_____

_____

20. A family member asks what sources you will use as you begin your employment search.

_____

_____

21. Your teacher asks you to describe the practices you must keep in mind regarding a résumé.

a. _____

b. _____

c. _____

d. _____

e. _____

f. _____

22. You are asked to list three steps to be taken when approaching an interview.

a. _____

b. _____

c. _____

23. You need to explain how you can make a new position more secure.

a. _____

b. _____

c. _____

d. _____

e. _____

24. A classmate asks you what are six ways to enhance your knowledge and education after certification.

a. _____

b. _____

c. _____

d. _____

e. _____

f. _____

True/False. Mark the following true or false by circling T or F.

25. T   F   At an interview, you should wait to be invited before sitting.

26. T   F   Body language is very important in conveying your interest in employment.

27. T   F   Ask for a job description to be sure you are qualified for the position being offered.

28. T   F   Mail your résumé after the interview.

29. T   F   Always thank the interviewer at the end of the interview.

30. T   F   Every interview should be viewed as a learning experience.

31. T   F   Nursing and medical literature are good sources of information about patient conditions.

32. T   F   A two-week notice should be given before leaving a job.

33. T   F   You should be positive in a resignation even if you are leaving a position because something upsetting has happened.

34. T   F   Always date and sign a letter of resignation.

Résumé Writing.

35. Practice writing a résumé. Be sure when you have finished to check it against the list of areas to be covered.

   a. your name, address, and telephone number

   b. your educational background

   c. your work history

   d. other experiences you have had

   e. references

   f. personal information about interests and activities

Practice Résumé

36. Using your résumé, complete the employment application on page 271.

37. In the space provided, practice writing a letter of resignation.

_____

(DATE)

Dear _____

It is necessary for me to leave my position as _____

(POSITION)

as of _____ . Working here at _____

(EFFECTIVE DATE OF RESIGNATION)   (FACILITY NAME)

has given me an opportunity to _____ .

I find I must leave because _____

(REASON FOR LEAVING)

Thank you for your understanding of my situation.

Sincerely,

_____

(YOUR NAME)

CLEARWATER GENERAL HOSPITAL
Application for Employment

1. Full Name: _____

   Last   First   Middle   Maiden

   _____
   Street and Number or Rural Route

   _____
   City, State and ZIP Code

   _____
   County   Telephone or nearest—Specify
   Social Security Number _____

2. Person to notify in case of emergency:
   Name _____
   Address _____

   _____
   Telephone _____
   Relationship _____

3. Education: List in this order—High School, College. You must give complete addresses. Also, please note if you did not graduate from high school whether or not you have a GED certificate.

School	Address	City	State	Year

4. Work or Vocational Experience: Give most recent first.

Name of Institution or Company	Complete Address	Type of Work	Dates

5. Have you ever been arrested for anything other than minor traffic violations? Yes ___ No ___
6. Are you now or have you been addicted to the use of alcohol or habit-forming drugs? Yes___ No___
7. References: Name three people who know your qualifications or who know your character. They must not be related to you.

   Name _____
   Address _____ Telephone _____

   Name _____
   Address _____ Telephone _____

   Name _____
   Address _____ Telephone _____

8. What are your reasons for wishing to work at this facility? Please answer this question in paragraph form on the back of this application.

PART 2

Student Performance Record

STUDENT PERFORMANCE RECORD

Your teacher will evaluate each procedure you learn and perform, but it will be helpful if you also keep a record so you will know which experiences you still must master.

PROCEDURE				Date	Satisfactory	Unsatisfactory
UNIT 12 Infection Control						
OBRA	📹	Procedure 1	Handwashing			
OBRA	📹	Procedure 2	Putting on a Mask			
OBRA	📹	Procedure 3	Putting on a Gown			
OBRA	📹	Procedure 4	Putting on Gloves			
OBRA	📹	Procedure 5	Removing Contaminated Gloves			
OBRA	📹	Procedure 6	Removing Contaminated Gloves, Mask, and Gown			
OBRA	📹	Procedure 7	Serving a Meal in an Isolation Unit			
OBRA	📹	Procedure 8	Measuring Vital Signs in an Isolation Unit			
OBRA	📹	Procedure 9	Transferring Nondisposable Equipment Outside of Isolation Unit			
	📹	Procedure 10	Specimen Collection from Patient in an Isolation Unit			
OBRA	📹	Procedure 11	Caring for Linens in an Isolation Unit			
	📹	Procedure 12	Transferring Patient to and from an Isolation Unit			
		Procedure 13	Opening a Sterile Package			
UNIT 14 Patient Safety and Positioning						
OBRA	📹	Procedure 14	Turning the Patient Toward You			
OBRA	📹	Procedure 15	Turning the Patient Away from You			
OBRA	📹	Procedure 16	Moving a Patient to the Head of the Bed			
OBRA		Procedure 17	Logrolling the Patient			

OBRA Indicates an essential OBRA procedure   📹 Indicates a video procedure

PROCEDURE				Date	Satisfactory	Unsatisfactory
UNIT 15 The Patient's Mobility: Transfer Skills						
OBRA	🔲	Procedure 18	Applying a Transfer Belt			
OBRA	🔲	Procedure 19	Transferring the Patient from Bed to Chair—One Assistant			
OBRA	🔲	Procedure 20	Transferring the Patient from Bed to Chair—Two Assistants			
OBRA	🔲	Procedure 21	Transferring the Patient from Chair to Bed—One Assistant			
OBRA	🔲	Procedure 22	Transferring the Patient from Chair to Bed—Two Assistants			
OBRA		Procedure 23	Independent Transfer, Standby Assist			
		Procedure 24	Transferring the Patient from Bed to Stretcher			
		Procedure 25	Transferring the Patient from Stretcher to Bed			
OBRA	🔲	Procedure 26	Transferring the Patient with a Mechanical Lift			
OBRA	🔲	Procedure 27	Transferring the Patient onto and off the Toilet			
OBRA		Procedure 28	Transferring the Patient into and out of the Bathtub			
		Procedure 29	Transferring the Patient into and out of a Car			
UNIT 16 The Patient's Mobility: Ambulation						
OBRA	🔲	Procedure 30	Assisting the Patient to Walk with a Cane and Three-Point Gait			
OBRA	🔲	Procedure 31	Assisting the Patient to Walk with a Walker and Three-Point Gait			
OBRA	🔲	Procedure 32	Assisting the Falling Patient			
UNIT 17 Body Temperature						
OBRA	🔲	Procedure 33	Measuring an Oral Temperature (Glass Thermometer			
OBRA		Procedure 34	Measuring Temperature Using a Sheath-Covered Thermometer			

PROCEDURE			Date	Satisfactory	Unsatisfactory
OBRA		Procedure 35 Measuring a Rectal Temperature (Glass Thermometer)			
OBRA		Procedure 36 Measuring an Axillary or Groin Temperature (Glass Thermometer)			
OBRA		Procedure 37 Measuring an Oral Temperature (Electronic Thermometer)			
OBRA		Procedure 38 Measuring a Rectal Temperature (Electronic Thermometer)			
OBRA		Procedure 39 Measuring an Axillary Temperature (Electronic Thermometer)			
OBRA		Procedure 40 Measuring a Tympanic Temperature			
OBRA		Procedure 41 Cleaning Glass Thermometers			

UNIT 18 Pulse and Respiration

OBRA		Procedure 42 Counting the Radial Pulse			
		Procedure 43 Counting the Apical-Radial Pulse			
OBRA		Procedure 44 Counting Respirations			

UNIT 19 Blood Pressure

OBRA		Procedure 45 Taking Blood Pressure			

UNIT 20 Measuring Height and Weight

OBRA		Procedure 46 Weighing and Measuring the Patient Using an Upright Scale			
OBRA		Procedure 47 Weighing the Patient on a Chair Scale			
OBRA		Procedure 48 Measuring Weight with an Electronic Wheelchair Scale			
OBRA		Procedure 49 Measuring and Weighing the Patient in Bed			

UNIT 21 Admission, Transfer, and Discharge

		Procedure 50 Admitting the Patient			
		Procedure 51 Transferring the Patient			
		Patient 52 Discharging the Patient			

PROCEDURE				Date	Satisfactory	Unsatisfactory
UNIT 22 Bedmaking						
OBRA	■	Procedure 53	Making a Closed Bed			
OBRA		Procedure 54	Opening the Closed Bed			
OBRA	■	Procedure 55	Making an Occupied Bed			
		Procedure 56	Making the Surgical Bed			
UNIT 23 Patient Bathing						
OBRA	■	Procedure 57	Assisting with the Tub Bath or Shower			
OBRA	■	Procedure 58	Bed Bath			
OBRA		Procedure 59	Partial Bath			
OBRA	■	Procedure 60	Female Perineal Care			
OBRA	■	Procedure 61	Male Perineal Care			
OBRA	■	Procedure 62	Hand and Fingernail Care			
OBRA		Procedure 63	Bed Shampoo			
OBRA	■	Procedure 64	Dressing and Undressing Patient			
UNIT 24 General Comfort Measures						
OBRA	■	Procedure 65	Assisting with Routine Oral Hygiene			
OBRA	■	Procedure 66	Assisting with Special Oral Hygiene			
OBRA		Procedure 67	Assisting Patient to Brush and Floss Teeth			
OBRA	■	Procedure 68	Caring for Dentures			
OBRA	■	Procedure 69	Backrub			
OBRA	■	Procedure 70	Shaving a Male Patient			
OBRA		Procedure 71	Daily Hair Care			
OBRA	■	Procedure 72	Giving and Receiving the Bedpan			
OBRA	■	Procedure 73	Giving and Receiving the Urinal			
OBRA	■	Procedure 74	Assisting with Use of the Bedside Commode			
UNIT 25 Nutritional Needs and Diet Modifications						
OBRA	■	Procedure 75	Assisting the Patient Who Can Feed Self			
OBRA	■	Procedure 76	Feeding the Dependent Patient			

PROCEDURE			Date	Satisfactory	Unsatisfactory
UNIT 26 Warm and Cold Applications					
	Procedure 77	Applying an Ice Bag			
	Procedure 78	Applying a Disposable Cold Pack			
	Procedure 79	Applying an Aquamatic K-Pad®			
	Procedure 80	Performing a Warm Soak			
	Procedure 81	Applying a Warm Moist Compress			
	Procedure 82	Assisting with Application of a Hypothermia Blanket			
UNIT 27 Assisting with the Physical Examination					
	Procedure 83	Assisting with a Physical Examination			
UNIT 28 the Surgical Patient					
	Procedure 84	Shaving the Operative Area			
	Procedure 85	Assisting Patient to Deep Breathe and Cough			
	Procedure 86	Performing Postoperative Leg Exercises			
OBRA	Procedure 87	Applying Elasticized Stockings			
	Procedure 88	Applying Elastic Bandage			
OBRA	Procedure 89	Assisting Patient to Dangle			
UNIT 30 Death and Dying					
OBRA	Procedure 90	Giving Postmortem Care			
UNIT 34 Subacute Care					
	Procedure 91	Changing a Gown on a Patient with a Peripheral Intravenous Line in Place			
UNIT 36 Respiratory System					
	Procedure 92	Refilling the Humidifier Bottle			
	Procedure 93	Collecting a Sputum Specimen			
UNIT 38 Musculoskeletal System					
OBRA	Procedure 94	Performing Range-of-Motion Exercises (Passive)			

PROCEDURE			Date	Satisfactory	Unsatisfactory
UNIT 39 Endocrine System					
	Procedure 95	Testing Urine for Acetone: Ketostix® Strip Test			
UNIT 40 Nervous System					
OBRA	Procedure 96	Caring for Eye Socket and Artificial Eye			
OBRA	Procedure 97	Applying a Behind-the-Ear Hearing Aid			
OBRA	Procedure 98	Removing a Behind-the-Ear Hearing Aid			
OBRA	Procedure 99	Applying and Removing an In-the-Ear Hearing Aid			
UNIT 41 Gastrointestinal System					
	Procedure 100	Collecting a Stool Specimen			
📹	Procedure 101	Giving a Soap Solution Enema			
📹	Procedure 102	Giving a Commercially Prepared Enema			
	Procedure 103	Inserting a Rectal Suppository			
	Procedure 104	Inserting a Rectal Tube and Flatus Bag			
UNIT 42 Urinary System					
📹	Procedure 105	Collecting a Routine Urine Specimen			
📹	Procedure 106	Collecting a Clean-Catch Urine Specimen			
	Procedure 107	Collecting a Fresh Fractional Urine Specimen			
	Procedure 108	Collecting a 24-Hour Urine Specimen			
	Procedure 109	Testing Urine with the HemaCombistix®			
OBRA 📹	Procedure 110	Routine Drainage Check			
📹	Procedure 111	Giving Indwelling Catheter Care			
📹	Procedure 112	Emptying a Urinary Drainage Unit			
📹	Procedure 113	Disconnecting the Catheter			
📹	Procedure 114	Applying a Condom for Urinary Drainage			
📹	Procedure 115	Connecting a Catheter to a Leg Bag			
📹	Procedure 116	Emptying a Leg Bag			

PROCEDURE	Date	Satisfactory	Unsatisfactory
UNIT 43 Reproductive System			
Procedure 117 Breast Self-Examination			
Procedure 118 Giving a Nonsterile Vaginal Douche			
UNIT 46 Pediatric Patient			
Procedure 119 Admitting a Pediatric Patient			
Procedure 120 Weighing the Pediatric Patient			
Procedure 121 Changing Crib Linens			
Procedure 122 Changing Crib Linens (Infant in Crib)			
Procedure 123 Measuring Temperature			
Procedure 124 Determining Heart Rate (Pulse)			
Procedure 125 Counting Respiratory Rate			
Procedure 126 Measuring Blood Pressure			
Procedure 127 Bottle-Feeding the Infant			
Procedure 128 Burping (Method A)			
Procedure 129 Burping (Method B)			
UNIT 47 Special Advanced Procedures			
Procedure 130 Testing for Occult Blood Using Hemoccult® and Developer			
Procedure 131 Testing for Occult Blood Using Hematest® Reagent Tablets			
Procedure 132 Collecting a Urine Specimen Through a Drainage Port			
Procedure 133 Giving Routine Stoma Care (Colostomy)			
Procedure 134 Routine Care of an Ileostomy (with Patient in Bed)			
UNIT 48 Response to Basic Emergencies			
Procedure 135 Adult CPR, One Rescuer			
Procedure 136 Adult CPR, Two-Person			
Procedure 137 Heimlich Maneuver—Abdominal Thrusts			

PROCEDURE		Date	Satisfactory	Unsatisfactory
OBRA Procedure 138 Assisting the Adult Who Has an Obstructed Airway and Becomes Unconscious				
Procedure 139 CPR for Infants				
Procedure 140 Obstructed Airway: Conscious Infant				
Procedure 141 Obstructed Airway: Unconscious Infant				
Procedure 142 CPR for Children, One Rescuer				
Procedure 143 Child with Foreign Body Airway Obstruction				

PART 3

Flashcards

abdoin/o	cephal/o
aden/o	cerebr/o
adren/o	chol/e
angi/o	chondr/o
arteri/o	col/o
arthr/o	cost/o
bronch/o	crani/o
card, cardi/o	cyst/o

head	abdomen
brain	gland
bile	adrenal gland
cartilage	vessel
colon, large intestine	artery
rib	joint
skull	bronchus, bronchi
bladder, cyst	heart

cyt/o	gloss/o
dent/o	hem, hema
derma	hemo, hemat
encephal/o	hepat/o
enter/o	hyster/o
erythr/o	ile/o
gastr/o	lapar/o
geront/o	laryng/o

tongue	cell
blood	tooth
blood	skin
liver	brain
uterus	small intestine
ileum	red
abdomen, loin, flank	stomach
larynx	old age

mamm/o	oophor/o
mast/o	ophthalm/o
men/o	oste/o
my/o	ot/o
myel/o	pharyng/o
nephr/o	phleb/o
neur/o	pneum/o
ocul/o	proct/o

ovary	breast
eye	breast
bone	menstruation
ear	muscle
pharynx	spinal cord bone marrow
vein	kidney
lung, air, gas	nerve
rectum	eye

psych/o	thorac/o
pulm/o	thym/o
rect/o	thyr/o
rhin/o	trache/o
salping/o	ur/o
splen/o	urethr/o
stern/o	urin/o
stomat/o	uter/o

chest	mind
thymus	lung
thyroid	rectum
trachea	nose
urine, urinary tract, urination	auditory (eustachian) tube, uterine (fallopian) tube
urethra	spleen
urine	sternum
uterus	mouth

ven/o	thromb/o
fibr/o	tox/o, toxic/o
glyc/o	a—
gynec/o	ante—
hydr/o	anti—
lith/o	bio—
ped/o	brady—
py/o	contra—

clot	vein
poison	fiber
without	sugar
before	woman
against, counteracting	water
life	stone
slow	child
against, opposed	pus

dys—	poly—
hyper—	pre—
hypo—	pseudo—
inter—	tachy—
intra—	—centesis
neo—	—genic
pan—	—gram
peri—	—logy

many	pain or difficulty
before	above, excessive
false	low, deficient
fast	between
puncture or aspiration of	within
producing, causing	new
record	all
study of	around

—lysis	—rrhagia
—megaly	—rrhea
—otomy	—scope
—pathy	—scopy
—penia	—stasis
—plegia	
—pnea	
—ptosis	

excessive flow	destruction
profuse flow, discharge	enlargement
examination instrument	incision
examination using a scope	disease
maintaining a constant level	lack, deficiency
	paralysis
	breathing, respiration
	falling, sagging, dropping down